BIG BOLD BEAUTIFUL

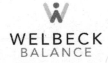

WELBECK
BALANCE

BIG BOLD BEAUTIFUL

The Soul-Seeker's Guide to Creating
an Empowered Purpose-Driven Life

Kate Taylor

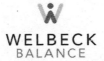

WELBECK
BALANCE

For the Disco Ball Crew
Let's get ready to shine.

ABOUT THE AUTHOR

Lover of disco balls, a bright red lip and more leopard print than is necessary, Kate Taylor isn't your average coach. She's a leading life and business empowerment coach, author, trainer and mentor; Master NLP practitioner; Qoya teacher, author and speaker; and creator of the Practical Magic Activation Deck – a life coach in a box.

She brings spark, magic and a bit of rock 'n' roll technicolour to her clients' lives. They call her the human dream-catcher, due to her mission to help them live a BIG, BOLD, BEAUTIFUL life. She's here to help you light up the fire in your heart and your belly, take up space, and create from your calling so that you can make a difference – not just to your world, but to THE world.

www.katetaylor.co
@katetaylorcreativeliving

Published in 2023 by Welbeck Balance
An imprint of Welbeck Non-Fiction Limited
Part of Welbeck Publishing Group
Offices in: London – 20 Mortimer Street, London W1T 3JW &
Sydney – Level 17, 207 Kent St, Sydney NSW 2000 Australia
www.welbeckpublishing.com

Design and layout © Welbeck Non-Fiction Ltd 2023
Text © Kate Taylor 2023

A CIP catalogue record for this book is available from the British Library.

ISBN
978-1-80129-260-3

Typeset by Lapiz Digital Services
Printed in Great Britain by CPI Group (UK) Ltd

10 9 8 7 6 5 4 3 2 1

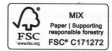

MIX
Paper | Supporting
responsible forestry
FSC® C171272

Note/Disclaimer
Welbeck encourages and welcomes diversity and different viewpoints. However, all
views, thoughts and opinions expressed in this book are the author's own and are not
necessarily representative of Welbeck Publishing Group as an organization. Welbeck
Publishing Group makes no representations or warranties of any kind, express or implied,
with respect to the accuracy, completeness, suitability or currency of the contents of this
book, and specifically disclaims, to the extent permitted by law, any implied warranties of
merchantability or fitness for a particular purpose and any injury, illness, damage, death,
liability or loss incurred, directly or indirectly from the use or application of any of the
information contained in this book. This book is solely intended for informational purposes
and guidance only and is not intended to replace, diagnose, treat or act as a substitute for
professional and expert medical and/or psychiatric advice. The author and the publisher
are not medical practitioners nor counsellors and professional advice should be sought
before embarking on any health-related programme.

Any names, characters, trademarks, service marks and trade names detailed in this book
are the property of their respective owners and are used solely for identification and
reference purposes. This book is a publication of Welbeck Non-Fiction, part of
Welbeck Publishing Group and has not been licensed, approved, sponsored or
endorsed by any person or entity.

Every reasonable effort has been made to trace copyright holders of material
produced in this book, but if any have been inadvertently overlooked the
publishers would be glad to hear from them.

CONTENTS

INTRODUCTION

Welcome, you wonderful soul seeker. Welcome to the beginning of this journey into living a BIG, BOLD, BEAUTIFUL life. I'm so glad you are here. We are about to embark on an adventure of a lifetime, and it honestly gives me the feels every time I know someone is opening the first pages of this book, curious about what lies ahead.

As a curious soul seeker, you're the kind of person I love spending time with – because you are ready to look at life in a different way. You are ready to take the things that may have been leaving you feeling a little "meh" around the edges, and find new possibilities to explore that feel much more "you-shaped". As you make your way through this seven-step guide to living a BIG, BOLD, BEAUTIFUL life, you are going on a voyage of discovery to find out more about yourself – what makes you tick, and what makes you feel alive – on both the inside, and the outside of your precious life. And ultimately, what gives you that fully fired up confidence to step away from a life of grey and into your life of full technicolour shine!

So, strap yourself in and get ready for the adventure of a lifetime that lifts you up and out of these pages, on a journey through seven steps beyond overwhelm and indecision and into an extraordinary, purpose-driven adventure.

WHAT IS A BIG, BOLD, BEAUTIFUL LIFE?

Before we delve on in, let's explore what living a BIG, BOLD, BEAUTIFUL life is all about. Now, your BIG, BOLD, BEAUTIFUL life is going to look different to mine, and mine is going to look different from that of the next person reading this book, but the principles are the same – they are the very foundations you will explore within these pages that, when implemented, become an approach for living life on your own terms. What you will learn will help you shift, grow and develop at each pivotal stage of your life, and every time you hot-step into something new.

BIG

Living a BIG life is about creating the kind of expansive dreams, visions and soul goals that make you fizz with excitement. The ones that stretch you beyond the realms of not just what is possible, but take you to where you might be a little bit afraid to speak out loud in case it does actually happen! Don't worry, you're not going to read this book and pack your life into two suitcases to go off on a wild adventure – unless that really is the thing on your vision board! No, living a BIG life is about taking stock of where you are now, and checking in. Checking in on what is good, and where it could be great. Checking in, and getting really honest, about where you might be holding yourself back, and where – and how – you are playing it safe trying to make everyone else happy, while you feel time slipping away from you as your fire and zest for life fizzles out.

What you are going to find within this book is going to disrupt how things are right now – in the best possible way – because it's only when we step off from the treadmill of the life that feels out of alignment that we can get the clarity to see what needs to change. And it's from this place that you can work out where you've had the volume turned down on your dreams and desires, and what is out there for you ... even if you don't know what that is yet. What's within these pages will help you explore what gets you activated and feeling alive, and figure out how you are going to turn up that dial on your boundless vision and vibrancy!

BOLD

Living a BOLD life is about having that BIG vision and taking up the space in your life to make it happen. It's about making the conscious decision to say goodbye to playing small or apologizing for being you. It's about ditching the role of the people pleaser, and stripping off the many masks you might be wearing right now, trying to make everyone else happy. It's about being *all you*, even if you've forgotten what that feels like – or if you never knew in the first place! Stepping into your BOLD life can be as gentle as it can be fierce; it can mean no fucks given and being an activist for what you believe makes the world a better place. It's about getting back to the essence of you, who you were before the world told you to be something else.

One thing is for sure – as you navigate what's within these pages, and what's within you that's ready to burst out of that chrysalis – you are invited to spread those BIG, BOLD, BEAUTIFUL wings of yours. It's time to call time on the curse of not feeling enough or worrying about being "too much". Basically, you're going to break up with the BS that's been running the show. Living BOLD means becoming more you than you've ever been before, and feeling powered up on the inside as you become unapologetically you. I hope you're ready, because I am!

BEAUTIFUL

Living a BEAUTIFUL life is about curating a life on your own terms, which positively impacts you, and those you love. It's about living a life that you've fallen deeply in love with and that loves you right back. It's about crafting a life and a living legacy that has full purpose and meaning. The kind that makes your heart skip a beat when you think about it. It's the life lived in joy and rich with contentment. One lived with compassion in your heart, and a story in your soul. It's the one where you take a moment and look around at what you've created and say to yourself, "I made this happen." Your BEAUTIFUL life reflects love both inward and outward toward the world, rather than being held down by the never-ending to-do lists or the "shoulds" that take the shine off. It's about looking out on each day and seeing the possibility of what lies ahead of you, rather than dreading what might happen, or hasn't happened yet.

Your BEAUTIFUL life is one of your own making. It's the one where you can come home to yourself any time you need to … because it is you. Sounds all kinds of delicious? It is, and it's ready and waiting for you to step into it.

YOUR VERSION OF YOUR BIG, BOLD, BEAUTIFUL LIFE

Everything you are going to explore within this guide is open for reflection, curiosity and discovery. As you delve and dive into the covers and concepts inside these pages, you will be invited to explore what is being activated within you, and how what is being shared relates to you. You are as unique as your fingerprints. So, too, is your BIG, BOLD, BEAUTIFUL LIFE. So, before we go any further, take a few minutes to journal on what a BIG, BOLD, BEAUTIFUL life means to you.

Let your heart and hand take the lead; there's no way you can do it wrong. Use these prompts as a starting point:

For me a BIG life is …

....

....

....

A BOLD life is …

....

....

....

A BEAUTIFUL life is …

....

....

....

This is a great place to start from – and to come back to – once you've been through the seven steps. That way you can reflect on what's shifted or grown on your pathway of potentiality.

LIVING YOUR BIG, BOLD, BEAUTIFUL LIFE IS A COMMITMENT

Reading this book isn't the secret sauce to getting everything you desire for your life and more. Living a BIG, BOLD, BEAUTIFUL life doesn't magically happen overnight. It's a voyage of discovery and adventure. I want to applaud you for stepping into this space – it takes courage and commitment to activate change. Living your BIG, BOLD, BEAUTIFUL life is something to commit to each and every day … sometimes, 100 times a day.

Living BIG, BOLD, BEAUTIFUL is a vibe. It's a check-in point, as much as it's a way of both becoming and being. You're evolving into the full essence of everything you are here to be, discovering more about yourself with every breath. And your *being* is your heart, beating life into the truth of who you are.

The BIG, BOLD, BEAUTIFUL path is not always the easiest road to travel. You will face fears and doubts along the way. Sometimes, those fears and doubts will show up on the faces of those who you spend time with. Sometimes, you will carry on because it feels too good not to. At other times you will wobble and wonder if you can really do it. Or you will be so sure of your direction of travel that your wobbles become your wins.

The path of self-awareness and self-discovery is exactly that — a path that is going to take you on a wild ride into the unknown. As you hop on board this epic ride, the one true thing to remember — and to remind yourself often — is that you have everything within you to make this happen.

So, before we buckle up for the ride, make a commitment to your BIG, BOLD, BEAUTIFUL life right now. Then keep yourself reminded of it every time fear and doubt jump in the passenger seat to try and throw you off course.

MAKING YOUR COMMITMENT …

Write out these words in your journal:

"I AM COMMITTING TO MY BIG, BOLD, BEAUTIFUL LIFE." Then sign and date it (bonus points for writing it out and displaying it somewhere you can see it every day).

HOW I CAME TO LIVE A BIG, BOLD, BEAUTIFUL LIFE

I haven't always lived a BIG, BOLD, BEAUTIFUL life. In fact, for quite a long time, life couldn't have been more different. Before becoming a life design and empowerment coach, who spends every day working with clients to help them find meaning and vibrancy in their purpose-driven BIG, BOLD, BEAUTIFUL lives, I was a stressed out, burnt out London ad executive having an existential crisis. Work hard and play hard was the prerequisite for every job I'd ever had, and I took on that identity. I wore it like a badge of honour. I followed a path based on what I thought success should look like. I wanted to make those in my life proud of me. But I was a hot mess over-achiever and felt like an imposter. From the outside everything looked perfect but on the inside I felt disconnected and dissatisfied.

While on this treadmill of hustle life hit hard. As I turned 30 I lost both of my parents and a close friend in an unlucky three years. This certainly shocked me into questioning life and every aspect of what I thought was expected of me. I realized I was living a half-life, simply going through the motions. At first I thought the dissatisfaction meant I just had to try harder. But that didn't work, because no matter the hours I put in, the pain of the grief I was trying to run away from was still there.

Such big losses leave something of an indelible question mark over everything you've ever thought to be true. Everything got thrown around like I had taken up life inside a clothes dryer. It made me wonder what a life really is — a joyful life, a fulfilled life, a rich life — not just one that goes through the motions waiting until retirement to kick back, sit back and relax.

This lesson was delivered in a less-than-subtle way, after losing my dad to a long and drawn-out battle with Parkinson's disease. Mum collapsed just three days after Dad went into a residential home. She was just six months into her retirement. Instead of enjoying her time, she died just four weeks after dad went into permanent care. It taught me a lot, loss always does, but most importantly, it taught me to pay attention.

Even though everything I was doing and working for looked great from the outside in, the truth was that I felt I was living a life that was no longer the right fit. The sense of "Is this really it?" wouldn't leave me alone. As much as I tried to think my way out of it my bumper car thoughts had me questioning everything. There was no amount of white wine that could help me find the answers. Trying to distract myself by working hard and playing harder than ever wasn't cutting it. I had been living inside my head 24/7 and I was disconnected. I had been trying to make everyone else happy but ended up making myself miserable.

And yet, something inside of me was stirring. Something kept tapping my shoulder and telling me that it was time to follow a different path. One that had meaning to it. One where I could find out who I really was at my core so I could help others to explore more of who they were.

PURPOSE WAS CALLING

I had to get curious and follow the breadcrumb trails to rediscover what I had pushed aside to pursue a "grown-up" identity. I was fascinated about what makes people tick, what makes us who we truly are, what makes us creative and who we truly want to be, and what gets in the way of that. I didn't have too far to go; I worked in a creative industry and my job was to get the best out of people – my clients, my teams. My own dissatisfaction was a strength. It got me questioning how I'd thought things were supposed to be. And once I questioned it in my life I saw it everywhere – the brilliant women around me apologizing and not taking up space because they lacked confidence. Being shot down if they voiced an opinion that went against the grain, or being told they were "too emotional" if they expressed dissatisfaction or frustration. Professional and personal versions of themselves were trying to have it all and make everyone else happy, losing who they were in the mix. I saw things that I could no longer un-see. This new fire had been lit, and my soul was fanning the flames, making me eager to find the "something more" in life.

Death had made life appear extraordinary. I was being invited on a journey of becoming and connecting beyond the logical mind. And this would be where I could make a positive difference.

What followed was an adventure to discover what living a BIG, BOLD, BEAUTIFUL life could be. This adventure took me down a path to becoming a life coach and master Neuro Linguistic Programming (NLP) practitioner. It took me away from a safe, comfortable life, to the jungles of Costa Rica to connect to my wise, wild and free self through a somatic movement practice called Qoya. My journey to discovery has forced me to question every aspect of life. I started to say YES to the adventure and NO to things that are no longer meant for me. It took huge courage and big risks, even when it was not clear they would work out. But this approach has unlocked so much inside of me and it continues to do so each and every day. I have breathed BIG, BOLD, BEAUTIFUL life into everything I do. And as a life design and empowerment coach I can help others to live their version of what a BIG, BOLD, BEAUTIFUL life means for them. It's an honour to be your guide on this adventure of a lifetime.

STARTING BEFORE YOU'RE READY

You don't have to be totally ready as you embark on this adventure with your BIG, BOLD, BEAUTIFUL life, but you do have to be willing to make a start. You don't have to throw everything away and do everything from scratch, but you do have to be curious about what is going on in your life that feels anything other than BIG, BOLD and BEAUTIFUL. The kind of curiosity that will serve you well throughout this journey is what led you to pick up this book in the first place.

You might be beyond ready to step away from the sea of confusion and overwhelm that seems to be creeping into every area of your life, or you might be in need of a big old lie down as you teeter on the edge of burnout.

PUT AN END TO OVERWHELM

I see you, and I've got you. You're not failing if you feel like you struggle to hold it together. And you're certainly not the only one who hasn't got their shit together, despite what you tell yourself. If you long to get back to that sparky, energetic version of yourself, you are not alone. If it feels like everything is on your shoulders, and that the idea of "having it all" has been mis-sold, it's because it has.

Life seems to get busier and more overwhelming. The boundaries between technology, life and work are blurred. And I'm going to hazard a guess that so are your own personal boundaries between what you think is expected of you, and what you take on.

COMBAT INDECISION

It might seem like you are at least 1,000 decisions ahead of everyone else around you in your life; it can all feel like it's just too much. This stress and busyness make it much harder to come home to the decisions you get to make on the things that feel true to you. Decision fatigue is real, and if you feel like you're not moving forward because you're scared of making the wrong choices, then decision fatigue could well be what's making it seem harder.

What's within this book isn't about creating endless choices. Living a BIG, BOLD, BEAUTIFUL life isn't all about doing more. In fact, much of the time it's about simplification. It's about finding a shortcut to fulfilment that feels true for you – beyond the noise and the overwhelm. It's about living an empowered life, embodying a truth that comes from within you, filling up every cell in your body.

BIG, BOLD and BEAUTIFUL is a call to rise for women who want to live empowered and embodied lives, questioning expectations and outdated obligations. And when you lead on the path for other women to do the same, you become a force to be reckoned with. You become dangerous in so many BIG, BOLD, BEAUTIFUL ways, and I'm here for it!

WHY I'M OBSESSED WITH DISCO BALLS
(AND WHY READING THIS BOOK MIGHT JUST MAKE YOU OBSESSED WITH THEM TOO!)

I have to confess to my obsession with disco balls! For me there is nothing more BIG, BOLD and BEAUTIFUL than throwing shapes under a disco ball on a great night out. The disco ball has become a totem for all things BIG, BOLD and BEAUTIFUL in my life and work.

I think of our hearts as a disco ball, made up of lots of tiny mirrors reflecting out the light of who we are to the world. Not all of the mirrors on the disco ball can reflect light all the time, so some of those tiny fragments of glass are in shadow. It's the same with you; you are light, shade and everything in between. Your stories, your experiences, your fuck-ups and your fabulousness. All of it is a reflection of all of you and how you are here to shine out your love and fullest self to the world.

Activating your disco ball heart through living a BIG, BOLD, BEAUTIFUL life gives you the permission to own all of you, in a way that is true to your own authentic experience, as well as the permission to step onto the dancefloor of your own precious life. Your only job is to light up your heart. Because when you are lit up, you help others to light up – friends, family, the community and beyond.

This is an invitation to light up the world by shining that disco ball heart of yours out into the world. It starts with you.

A QUICK WORD ABOUT YOUR (SOUL) PURPOSE ... NO BIGGIE!

Before we get started on the seven steps to living a BIG, BOLD, BEAUTIFUL life, let's talk about the quest for purpose. It wasn't something I was aware of before, but it is something I very much live my life by, each and every day.

Many people come to this voyage of discovery at pivotal points in their lives because they are searching for something to make life make sense. Lots of my clients come to me feeling like they are stuck at a crossroads, and that without a clear direction of travel, life just feels like Groundhog Day. They feel that if they can find purpose, then life will become a carpet ride of fulfilment and flow – that state of being in enjoyment and energetic alignment to a sense of being exactly where you are supposed to be, and heading in a clear direction on the path you are meant to be on.

Some of this is true, and some of it isn't. For starters, purpose isn't something you find – it's not lost down the back of the sofa waiting for you to pull it out with the fluff and old coins. Purpose is something that is already within you. It's something that *reveals itself to you* when you embark on your voyage of discovery and self-awareness.

Your purpose is made up of all facets of you. It's what makes your disco ball heart shine. It is the golden thread that weaves through your experiences, your stories, your gifts, your skills, your identity, your personality, your attributes … your wild self-expression! And when you blend this with your triumphs, challenges and tribulations it becomes possible for you to shine a light on all of the hidden gems that make up your disco ball heart.

WHAT IS SOUL PURPOSE?

Your soul purpose is the true essence of who you are at a soul level and how you bring that into your life through your calling, getting in step with everything that you are, and everything that you are here to do.

This book and the steps and guidance within, will take you on a journey to reveal more of your light, through your connection to your soul's purpose.

THE SEVEN STEPS TO LIVING A BIG, BOLD, BEAUTIFUL LIFE
(AND HOW TO USE THIS BOOK)

This guide will take you on a seven-step adventure to design and create a BIG, BOLD, BEAUTIFUL and purpose-driven life.

You will find that the steps become tools for life that you can come back to as and when you are setting out on a new project or venture. It's also really great to revisit the steps at the beginning of a new year, or around your birthday, when you might want to create some new intentions and goals for the year ahead. They also really come into their own any time you are feeling at a crossroads, or stuck in a rut, and you want a kickstart to get yourself up and at it for a BIG, BOLD, BEAUTIFUL life.

The steps are split into two parts:

✓ In the first part (STEPS ONE and TWO) you will create your vision, soul goals and action plan. Your vision and soul goals form the direction of travel for your BIG, BOLD, BEAUTIFUL life, and you'll also work on curating focus and an aligned action plan of how to go about getting what it is you truly desire. These two foundational steps will set the tone for what you are creating.
✓ The second part (STEPS THREE to SEVEN) equips you with the energetic and practical tools you need to make your journey a reality. These steps are the support act for your BIG, BOLD, BEAUTIFUL vision and soul goals.

After you have worked your way through this guide fully once, you can revisit any step along your BIG, BOLD, BEAUTIFUL journey as and when you need that support.

Here's an overview of each step:

STEP ONE: CREATE THE VISION (FOR YOUR BIG, BOLD, BEAUTIFUL LIFE)

This is where you will set the destination in the sat nav for your BIG, BOLD, BEAUTIFUL life. You'll do this through establishing your vision, and creating soul goals that align with this vision and core values, so that the change you are creating comes from the inside out.

STEP TWO: FIND YOUR FOCUS

Here, we take your BIG, BOLD, BEAUTIFUL vision and soul goals and help them come to fruition by creating simple and sustainable actions. Importantly, STEP TWO will help you avoid immediate overwhelm and over-complication, by keeping things simple, effective and moving. You will explore spiritual and strategic ways to work with your energy. Honestly, this step will become your best friend, helping you move away from procrastination and toward aligned and focused action.

STEP THREE: BUST BEYOND RESISTANCE

The first of the tools you'll need on your journey, we start by looking at how to break through the inevitable resistance that hits every time you step out of your comfort zone. You will explore how resistance shows up for you, and the mind-body connection that both fuels and busts resistance, so that you can move beyond any stuck energy that could hold you back from taking action.

STEP FOUR: DIAL UP YOUR BIG, BOLD, BEAUTIFUL ENERGY

Focusing on the energy that will support and sustain you as you walk and dance through your BIG, BOLD, BEAUTIFUL journey, this step delves deeper into the mind-body connection. You will explore body wisdom, and how your superhighway connector – the vagus nerve – powers up your body's intelligence centres. You will learn to connect with the wonderful wisdom that fires the fuel that connects you and helps you to become a vibrational match for your BIG, BOLD, BEAUTIFUL vision and soul goals.

STEP FIVE: CREATE A SELF-EMPOWERMENT TOOLKIT

This is the confidence and empowerment booster you need to give you the courage, strength and resolve to move forward and take action toward your BIG, BOLD, BEAUTIFUL soul goals. It puts the pep into each and every step. You will explore how to create rocking self-belief that will support you, not just for your soul goals, but for life. And how you can ultimately rock out with your socks out, and put the BOLD in your BIG, BOLD, BEAUTIFUL into your vision and goals, by creating the conditions that boost your confidence and self-esteem.

STEP SIX: HONOUR YOUR SELF-CARE

You will find wellbeing principles woven throughout the seven steps. That's because when working toward your goals it can be all too easy to tip over into overwhelm and burnout (which is the antithesis of a BIG, BOLD, BEAUTIFUL life!). STEP SIX is your definitive guide to creating the conditions that support your actions as you take the steps on your BIG, BOLD, BEAUTIFUL vision quest. You will explore ways to take care of your mind, body and soul with easy-to-implement wellbeing and self-care tools that help you activate that glorious disco ball heart of yours.

STEP SEVEN: HARNESS THE POWER OF SELF-CELEBRATION

At the crescendo of BIG, BOLD, BEAUTIFUL it's time to fire up the glitter confetti cannons and pop the champagne cork to celebrate the journey you've taken throughout this book. You will explore the power of celebration, and how it creates momentum and motivation, bringing your BIG, BOLD, BEAUTIFUL vision into brilliant being.

BIG, BOLD, BEAUTIFUL BREAKOUT RITUALS

In between each step there's an opportunity to anchor your BIG, BOLD, BEAUTIFUL experience with seven BIG, BOLD, BEAUTIFUL BREAKOUT rituals. These are beautiful spiritual practices, and grounded rituals for life that I have gathered as part of my own BIG, BOLD, BEAUTIFUL journey. I love to share them in my practices and teaching. The rituals shared in these pages will honour each step of your progress through this BIG, BOLD, BEAUTIFUL journey. They will give you a chance to pause, breathe, honour and reflect on your journey through this guide.

OK, are you ready to get started? I know I am. Let's go!

STEP ONE

CREATE THE VISION
(for your BIG, BOLD, BEAUTIFUL life)

Like all journeys the first step is key because it sets the tone and the pace for the entire adventure. In fact, without this one, you're going to keep going around in circles and wondering why you're not getting anywhere!

STEP ONE on the adventure of your BIG, BOLD, BEAUTIFUL life starts with creating the map for where you are going through creating your BIG, BOLD, BEAUTIFUL VISION. Your vision is the foresight, the spark, the dream. It creates clarity on what you want your life to be. This vision can come from something specific you want to create such as starting a new project, changing your career, or building a heart-centred business. Or it can be more general – the way you live your life, creating a new way of living that you feel would serve you well. This is where you get to paint the picture of your ideal life and bring it into technicolour in the here and now, with your intention painting the beautiful scenery, and what you take action on the delicious detail.

This might be the first time you've ever had the chance to be in true co-creation with what comes next. It may be – or it may feel like – the 100th. When you are in co-creation, you are able to connect and collaborate with all parts of yourself for a rounded perspective of your life – like working with your full energetic team. Your vision is the opportunity to have a say in what you want (and what you don't want) for your life. It's a chance to get clear on the direction of travel. You're setting the destination and making sure it's the right destination for you!

Through this step you will set the foundations for what you are bringing into being in all areas of your BIG, BOLD, BEAUTIFUL life from this point forward. It's where you will activate energetically aligned anchor points that you can keep coming back to on this adventure of creating your BIG, BOLD, BEAUTIFUL life. Because believe me when I say there will be twists and there will be turns, and sometimes you will throw yourself off-course completely ... but when you have an anchored, embodied vision to come back to, you can't go wrong.

You are going to carry out an energetic stock check of where you are right now, and what's brought you to this place, before you get to making plans and creating a BIG, BOLD, BEAUTIFUL vision of how you wish your life to be. All too often we want to skip to the good bit of creating shiny new opportunities, before we've taken time to see what isn't working, and what we want to change about that. It's important to make sure you're not dropping those heavy rocks into your backpack as you set out on the journey ahead! Conversely, if you are so ready for a big shift out of a rut or challenging time, you need to make sure that you're not throwing out all the good things too.

And then we're going to get into it: you are going to discover how to create BIG, BOLD, BEAUTIFUL soul goals that help you create a full-bodied, energetically aligned, sensory experience of the future you're creating, and bring it with a shebang into the present moment.

I love, love, love this step because it brings all the vibes into play. It creates an inevitability of being in alignment and a super-charged partnership between you and yourself on all levels of mind, body and soul. Creating your vision map powers up your BIG, BOLD, BEAUTIFUL soul goals, which are the marker points that spark expansion in all areas of your life. It's a powerful tool you will be able to pull out of your box of tricks every time you are ready to start a new adventure.

Within this step there is guidance, coaching exercises and activations for you, to kickstart what you are bringing into being. You can either write directly in the book or take it over to a journal so you can come back and replay the step any time you wish.

As with everything as you go on this BIG, BOLD, BEAUTIFUL voyage of discovery, allow yourself to be in the energy of openness, exploration and curiosity.

IN STEP ONE YOU WILL:

✓ *Get intentional* by activating the power of intention and being clear on what you're doing before you set out doing it!

✓ *Carry out an energetic stock check* as you learn to review and reflect on where you are now and understand what to say "goodbye" to and what you want to say "hello" to in your BIG, BOLD, BEAUTIFUL life.

✓ *Follow your inner compass* by finding your values so they become your guiding light on your BIG, BOLD, BEAUTIFUL vision quest, providing alignment at all times.

✓ *Create BIG, BOLD, BEAUTIFUL goals with soul* when you find out what they are and why they are super-powered compared to normal goal setting.

✓ *Create an Expansive Vision Map* that takes in a 360 view of your life to create expansion in all areas.

✓ *Create an anchored embodied sensory experience,* by energetically imprinting your future in the present moment, to bring your vision into being.

I hope you're ready because this is about to get BIG, BOLD and freaking BEAUTIFUL!

GETTING INTENTIONAL

"Intentions compressed into words enfold magical power."
Deepak Chopra

Your intention charges up the energy in the hopes, dreams and desires you are going to pour into the BIG, BOLD, BEAUTIFUL vision and soul goals you are about to create. I like to think of intentions as the ultimate energetic power source, starting the engine on what you are creating, before you've even put pen to paper or started putting your goals into action. Intention gives purpose and the inspiration or motivation to make those BIG, BOLD, BEAUTIFUL ideas and dreams come to life. Without vision and intention you set off on a new path without any understanding of your destination and the kind of journey you want to have.

The way I think about creating intention is by considering how I want to feel in any given moment. It's not just focused on an outcome, but on how the journey to that outcome feels. Your intention sets the energetic tone for your BIG, BOLD, BEAUTIFUL journey – your inner desire to create your outer world.

It's a vibe.

For example, when I set out on the journey to write this book the goal was to get a specific number of words written, then get it published and into your hands. However, my intention was to have the BIGGEST, BOLDEST and most BEAUTIFUL experience doing it. I wanted to feel relaxed, connected and in flow, with the energy of living a BIG, BOLD, BEAUTIFUL life. So, I would take myself off to beautiful locations in vibrant places to do that.

THE DIFFERENCE BETWEEN SETTING GOALS AND DECIDING ON INTENTIONS

I think of goals and intentions as what I would call "Practical Magic": where there is the existence of both a practical and "magical" approach to creating your BIG, BOLD, BEAUTIFUL vision. When you blend the spiritual (whatever that means to you) with the soulful and the strategic you can create true alchemy in all areas of your life. This spiritual, soulful and strategic approach is woven into everything you will find within these pages, and when it comes to creating powerfully connected goals and intentions for your BIG, BOLD, BEAUTIFUL life.

Let's explore more …

GOALS are **the known/logical sense** – the **PRACTICAL.**

- Goals are focused on the future.
- Goals are a destination or a specific achievement.
- Goals are external – what you want to be, to do and to have – the job title, the salary, the house, the car … They are the physical manifestation of your vision.

INTENTIONS are the **felt/sensory/embodied experiences** – the **MAGIC.**

- Intentions are the feeling that carries that energy into being.
- Intentions are in the present moment.
- Intentions are lived each day, regardless of achieving the goal or destination.
- Intentions are about your relationship with yourself and others.

EXERCISE

SET INTENTIONS FOR YOUR BIG, BOLD, BEAUTIFUL LIFE

Start by getting clear on how you want to feel as you set off on this path of creating your BIG, BOLD, BEAUTIFUL life. Here's some simple intention setting prompts for you to tune in to ...

What are three words that describe what you hope to experience over the next 6-12 months? E.g., fulfilled, inspired, confident, content, motivated, creative, empowered, happy, brave, free ...

....

What do those three words look like to you? E.g., When I have confidence I am able to do the things I've always wanted to do. When I am motivated I seek opportunities with energy and purpose.

....

....

....

How will you know when you've got them? What will you be experiencing that lets you know your intentions are alive? E.g., I will feel full of purpose and know exactly what I'm doing. Opportunities will come my way.

....

....

....

What will a BIG, BOLD, BEAUTIFUL life feel like for you? E.g., I am able to explore opportunities in life that I have always wanted to. I feel full of excitement about the possibilities that lie ahead of me.

....

....

....

In what area(s) of your life would you most like to feel this way? E.g., sense of self, purpose, relationships, family, money, work, home ...

....

....

....

These intentions are your energetic alignment as you navigate your BIG, BOLD, BEAUTIFUL path. We will explore how to connect and anchor these feelings to your soul goals to create an embodied sensory experience later on in this step, but first, let's carry out an energetic stock check to see where you are right in this moment – an important step before creating soul goals.

CARRYING OUT AN ENERGETIC STOCK CHECK

To know where you're going with your BIG, BOLD, BEAUTIFUL life you've got to know where you've come from. Knowing what you want to create over the next 12 months – or however long you want to take to bring your BIG, BOLD, BEAUTIFUL plans into play – means taking a look in the rearview mirror to see what's come before. This energetic stock check helps you connect to what keeps you motivated and what could hold you back. It's powerful to honour all of the lessons and rich information it provides.

It's all too easy to rush ahead getting super-excited about the possibilities of something, anything, that might be different to how it is now. The tendency is to "resolve" or "fix" what's not working in your life right now, without understanding what's underneath any of it. It quickly becomes a game of playing smash and grab and trying to change everything in one go.

It's important to be discerning, so that you don't lump the whole experience of, say, the last 12 months together into one bundle.

Our brains take in over 32GB of information each and every day. If we were trying to live our lives, make plans, review yesterday's highlights and fuck-ups, blink, breathe, scroll, work, think about what's for dinner and plan the next year of our BIG, BOLD, BEAUTIFUL life all in one go, we'd most likely fall over, or melt our brains. (This is not a proven scientific fact!) If you also tried to process all your emotions and triggers in one go, you would go into a sensory meltdown, so your brain filter deletes, distorts or generalizes information to make things make sense.

DELETING

Deleting means deleting information or hiding it from plain sight. Imagine if you had to remember how to take every action you took in one day – from breathing, to blinking, buying groceries, and changing the world – it would be too much to take on! It's the same over a week, a month, a year and a lifetime of experiences. The mind will delete things it considers irrelevant or not useful, so that it can focus.

Deleting examples:
"That didn't work out for me. I am a failure."
"I wasn't clever/talented/experienced/creative enough to make it work."

"I am just not good at X, Y or Z."
"I didn't do anything of any merit last year."

DISTORTING

Distorting means anything from exaggerating something that has (or hasn't) happened to going from a fear to full-on disaster movie in one fell swoop! We have an incredible ability to catastrophize in our imagination. It's like the mind has a one-track course focused on some of the more negative aspects of your life, and will show you a bleak outlook. You will tell yourself there are limited options based on the distorted information your mind is presenting to you.

Distorting examples:
"There's no-one to help me. I don't have any support."
"I'm useless with money."
"No-one will want to work with me."
"I can never make it work."
"I'm just no good at making relationships stick."

GENERALIZING

Generalizing is when your brain looks for patterns and conclusions about your life and the world around you. You will find yourself using catch-all terms such as "always", "never", "everyone", "everything". This is a particular challenge when it comes to making some positive strides forward, because you are literally pitting yourself against the world and telling yourself why you can't make things work, or why everything around you is setting you up for failure.

Generalizing examples:
"Everyone has got their shit together other than me."
"I need to do this before I run out of time."

"I have to do everything."

"There's no point in me doing that because it never works out."

"Good things don't happen to people like me."

Left unchecked this deletion, distortion and generalization completely skews your view of things that you've done and achieved, that could help you. Instead, you will find "evidence" of all the things you're rubbish at, because your ego is trying to stop you from making any glaring howlers. So, you carry around the crappy stuff with you when you are trying to do new things. These beliefs become statements that you tell yourself. They will put the brakes on anything you are trying to create in your BIG, BOLD, BEAUTIFUL life.

While it may seem that deletion, distortion and generalization may not be the best breeding ground for helping you make BIG, BOLD, BEAUTIFUL strides forward, with awareness it's possible to work with them. You can challenge the narratives that don't serve you and change up the stories and inner dialogue.

Getting underneath this, and understanding what you are saying "goodbye" to, will help you find ways to release yourself from any stories or situations. It'll help you to make sure they're not hitching a ride as you make your moves forward. You also get the opportunity to welcome what you want more of in your BIG, BOLD, BEAUTIFUL life by giving gratitude and inviting in – both energetically and consciously – more of what lights you up. The aim is that you are fuelled by the energy that will keep you going, rather than having to constantly navigate the stuff that will hold you back.

This journalling exercise is a really useful way to figure out what you want to welcome and turn your back on over the coming months.

EXERCISE

ENERGETIC STOCK CHECK
JOURNALLING PROMPTS

Take a few moments to reflect on these journalling prompts. Be curious about what comes up. You will find self-empowerment tools and exercises for working on powering up your self-belief later on, in STEP FIVE.

I'm using 12 months as a reference point but you can use these review and reflect questions as a monthly reflection too:

Looking back at this time last year ...

What was going on in your life?

....

....

What did you want the months that followed to be about for you? (i.e. what were your hopes and dreams last year?)

....

....

What has changed since then?

....

....

What has stayed the same?

....

....

List three big achievements from the last year:

1 ....

2 ....

3 ....

What did you learn about yourself as a result of these achievements?

....

....

What were some of your happiest, most fulfilling moments from last year?

....

....

What learnings can you take from this?

....

....

What have been some of the biggest challenges you've had over the last year?

....

....

What learnings can you take about your creativity, strength and resilience from these challenges?

....

....

What are you most grateful for about the things you've done and experienced in the last 12 months?

....

....

What are you ready to say goodbye to from the last 12 months?

....

....

What will saying goodbye to help you create space for?

....

....

On completing your energetic stock check, take some time to reflect on what you've gained awareness of ahead of creating your soul goals a little further on in this step.

FINDING YOUR WHY & YOUR VALUES

Now you've reflected on what's in the rearview mirror, it's time to get clear on what kind of fuel you've got in the tank that will help drive you forward. This is all about getting clear on what's important to you by uncovering your core values.

Your core values are generally one-word activation points that stir something within you, guide you internally and help you make sense of the world. They are your inner compass, your North Star; they will energetically pull you when you are in alignment with them, and repel you if you're not. They are essentially the things that are so important to you, you would live and die by them, such as "freedom", "love", "integrity", "equality", "compassion", etc. Without living by your values, you live a life that is only half-touched in terms of depth, connection and self-awareness.

Your core values are as unique to you as your fingerprints. You might find other people who have similar core values to you. You will love hanging out with them but only you have your lived experience. Understanding what drives you, and what's important to you, helps you express how you feel about the world and how you desire to navigate your way through life. Once you know them, you can't un-know them – they give you an amazing guidance system to live by, playing a big part in living on purpose.

Values do change over time. The values that you have as a teenager are naturally going be different from the values you have in your twenties, thirties, forties and fifties. So carrying out a values elicitation exercise, to help you to figure out what your values are right now, is a great checking in point to make sure that the vibes you're working on in your BIG, BOLD, BEAUTIFUL life are still meant for you.

They are a feeling, a sense, a vibe, because they come from the very essence of what's within you. You will find that if you know your values, it becomes easier and quicker to understand when you're out of alignment or off-track, so you can course-correct. This is where you can connect to your intuitive sense, or be guided by your own inner compass. Connecting to your intuition helps you to activate the answers that are within you. It's from here that you can take the most empowered actions, because only you can be guided to make decisions and actions based on what is true for you. It also eases the overwhelm of doubt and decision fatigue that comes from searching everywhere outside of yourself. You can find a million and one opinions and options by looking around you, but when you are tuned in to your values, it's a guidance system that never steers you on the wrong path, or down a path that isn't meant for you.

Here's an example: Think about the times in your life when you were making a decision and it didn't feel quite right – maybe it was a job opportunity that seemed great on paper. Logic said, "This is a good decision, because look at the money, the benefits and the opportunity ..." But something niggled away at you. It just didn't feel right. Maybe it was a sense or a feeling. Maybe some of the things the company did, or the way they seemed to treat people, didn't sit right. Maybe it was some of the language they used when speaking about people. Your internal guidance system will have been flashing warning signs that the way they operate was completely out of alignment with your core values of integrity, compassion and equality.

Head over to the next exercise to carry out a values elicitation exercise to explore what your core values are, and what's truly important to you. These will show up all the way through your soul goals, so it's the perfect opportunity to get the clarity on them before you create your BIG, BOLD, BEAUTIFUL vision map.

EXERCISE

DISCOVER YOUR CORE VALUES

Here's a simple values elicitation exercise to help you find your top three core values. Write a list of ten words below. To get yours, breathe deeply and go with what comes up. You may find words pop up like popcorn! Write them down, even if they don't seem to make logical sense just yet. Don't overthink it, simply go with what comes up.

Questions to ask yourself to find your core values:

- What is important to me? (E.g., creativity, autonomy)
- What's important to me in my life? (E.g., friendships, health)
- What would I want someone to know about me, or say about me as a person? (E.g., integrity, kindness)
- What would I feel upset about if it wasn't in my life? (E.g., love, sense of belonging)
- What was missing when I've felt uncomfortable in a job, or relationship? (E.g., empathy, opportunity)
- What do I really value in friendships or relationships? (E.g., fun, trust)

MY CORE VALUES

.... ☐

.... ☐

.... ☐

.... ☐

.... ☐

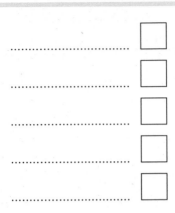

Now, looking at the list of core values above, number them from 10-1 in order of what is most important to you, with 10 being the least important, and then 9 the next.

- Check in on number 9 by asking yourself – Is this more or less important than 10? If it's more important, then keep it at 9. If it's less so, then swap them over.
- Put an 8 next to the value you believe is your number 8.
- Check in on 8 by asking yourself – is this more or less important than 9? If it's more important, then keep it at 8. If it's less so, then swap them over.
- Continue with 7, 6, 5, 4, 3, 2 and then 1.

The values with 1, 2 and 3 next to them are your top three values.

Once you have them, go back over them and connect to how you feel about your top three values. How do they feel in your body? Where do you feel them in your body? Do you feel them in your heart and your gut? Try them on for size. If you were wearing an outfit made up of these values, how would you feel going out into the world?

If they feel true for you, then write them out somewhere you can check in with them often. I have my top three values written on sticky notes in a place I can see them on a regular basis. I connect with them every time a potential new opportunity comes my way and my brain gets like an over-eager puppy. This makes sure that what I'm about to embark on is true and aligned for me.

As you start forming your BIG, BOLD, BEAUTIFUL soul goals and your vision map, it's important to ensure your values are honoured, otherwise you can spend a lot of time doing things for the sake of doing, rather than being in alignment to what's of true value to you.

CONNECTING TO THE ENERGETIC LANGUAGE OF EXPANSION VS. CONTRACTION

All of this work on your core values is the preparation for creating a BIG, BOLD, BEAUTIFUL life. To do this well you also need to use empowered language to add rocket-fuel to what you are creating.

Language is an ultimate power-source – what you speak, what you write, your inner dialogue, even your body language. It all creates energy at mind, body and soul level, which can either be expansive or contractive for the BIG, BOLD, BEAUTIFUL goals you are creating.

Think about words that might create soul expansion – joy, contentment, achievement, abundance; as opposed to words that could cause contraction – fear, loss, failure, debt. The energy these words create causes a physical response within the subconscious, your nervous system and your body, to either repel or magnetize. It's why affirmations are so powerful, because when you input positive and powerful language and energetic statements into your subconscious mind, body and nervous system, everything comes online to give a power-up boost in your energetic systems. Using the power of language and expansive energy, you can create super-charged, energetically aligned goals that move you toward what you want and away from what you don't want.

Of course, we're all wired differently. Some of us naturally move toward, and some naturally move away from where we want to go. It doesn't mean that there's anything wrong with you if you naturally move away from; it's just that you make sure you're flipping the scripts and creating a move toward goals using empowered language.

Examples of move away from vs. move toward empowered language flips include:

"Making sure I don't get into debt," (move away from) becomes "Managing my finances with ease and being in a financial overflow," (move toward).

"I need to make sure I don't make the same mistakes as last time and end up in a job I hate," (move away from) becomes "I have learned from all of my experiences and take them with me to ensure I am in a job that motivates and stimulates me," (move toward).

Try flipping the script on three examples of your own move away from and move toward goals.

Move away from   Move toward

.... → ....

.... → ....

.... → ....

While your "move away from" may sometimes be the driving factor, flipping the script on your language and establishing your "move toward" will create inspiring, motivational and sustainable BIG, BOLD, BEAUTIFUL goals.

So, let's get to it – it's time for the main event – creating your BIG, BOLD, BEAUTIFUL soul goals!

CREATING BIG, BOLD, BEAUTIFUL GOALS WITH SOUL

OK, this is where you are going to plug your BIG, BOLD, BEAUTIFUL destination into the sat nav. If you don't have a clear idea of where you're going and the map to get there, you're likely to get lost and take costly detours while burning a lot of fuel, only to arrive a lot later than you intended. And if you start out with what you think you should be doing, which is out of line with your values, it's going to send you on the wrong road entirely! Creating powerful and aligned goals that work for you on every level of your life, means you won't spend all your time, effort and energy going down a path, only to find it's not where you want to be.

You've figured out what's important to you, by nailing down your core values. How can you start to create a life plan that's aligned with those values? By setting goals. And not just goals, but goals with soul … Let's get to it!

SETTING GOALS WITH SOUL

A goal shoots an arrow into your future. Goals are fundamental whenever you are setting out to creating a positive change in your life. Traditional goal setting tends to be based on the external things you want to bring into being: the practical things you want to be, do and have, such as job title, salary, business success, etc. BIG, BOLD, BEAUTIFUL soul goals are aligned to your values and how you are making a positive impact on the world, woven with the golden thread of presence, vibing with intention and dripping with purpose.

Soul goals are super-powered goals. They weave your intention and your desires together to create tangible and specific outcomes that show you that you are hop, skipping and jumping in step with your soul, on the way to living your BIG, BOLD, BEAUTIFUL life. They are actions with meaning.

BIG, BOLD, BEAUTIFUL soul goals are about being in alignment with your deep sense of purpose, passion, meaning and calling. If the idea of this already feels like it's a lot to get right, then don't worry! It is most beautiful in its simplicity, and because it's coming from within you, there's no way you can do it wrong.

There is something of an art and a science to creating truly empowering BIG, BOLD, BEAUTIFUL goals that fill the very essence of your soul. You are going to get clear on what you want to have, just like you explored with your "move toward" and "move away from" when you were figuring out your core values.

THE SMART WAY TO CREATE GOALS

There are various ways of goal setting. One of the most common is SMART goals, which help you to create a specific action-orientated goal that gets you a result.

Specific/Significant: Your goal is precise and clearly defined; it has specificity and detail to it. It feels important. Your goal provides a clear instruction for the brain to follow and will help you know when you've got what you worked for.

Measurable/Meaningful: Because you've been specific with your goal, you will be able to demonstrate when you've achieved it. You will be able to measure your success and it will be quantifiable. The results of your goal will have meaning in your life.

Achievable/Attainable: Your goal is realistic. It is something that will be attainable within the realms of what you can create. It is achieved as a result of the actions you take.

Relevant/REALLY BLOODY GOOD!: Your goal relates to you and your life, and it feels like a motivating factor in your life.

Time-bound: Your goal will have a start and end date. You will create this goal within a certain timeframe, i.e., one month, six months, a year.

Here's an example of SMART goal setting

Specific/Significant: I'm going to carry out a project at work, which focuses on inclusion and sustainability, to empower marginalized groups within our customer base.

Measurable/Meaningful: I will present it to my team within the next three months. This will be a workshop style session, where we can create some positive things to work on. I truly believe in this project, as it aligns with my values of integrity, compassion and causing no harm.

Achievable/Attainable: I will interview five customers per week, over the next four weeks. This feels doable if I carve out one day per week to do it.

Relevant/REALLY BLOODY GOOD!: This project will give me something creative and empowering to focus on within my job. It will create opportunities for me in the future.

Time-bound: I will start the research for the interviews on Monday and get them booked in with selected customers by the end of next week.

SMART goal summary

A SMART goal can look like this ...

"I will carry out a project at work that focuses on inclusion and sustainability. It will empower marginalized customers. I will present this in a workshop to the team in three months' time. I will interview 20 customers in total and carve out one day per week over the next four weeks to gather the data. This will make a positive contribution to the company and my career; it will motivate me to do more."

I love SMART goals. They can be used in all scenarios for a super-practical way to set things in motion. They work when approached with logic, planning and clear direction. So, they're perfect when you need to get focused and get shit done. They are the friend who is brilliant at planning an evening out and taking care of all the details. That's great, you have a pleasant enough time ...

And then there's the friend who doesn't just plan an evening and take care of all the details ... They create the kind of memories and experiences that you will never, ever forget!

Enter BIG, BOLD, BEAUTIFUL soul goals. These are so much more than just getting-things-done goals. Soul goals take what you want to be, do and have, add truth and heart, and deliver on purpose. This is where you get to the juice of creating BIG, BOLD, BEAUTIFUL soul goals and make the manifestation of what you are putting out into the world a grounded experience.

To get your BIG, BOLD, BEAUTIFUL soul goals, you can use the five Ps of goal setting:

1. **Present tense:** Writing goals in the present tense brings them into the now, as if they are already here. They are "I am" and "I have" statements.
2. **Positive:** Harnessing your "move toward" energy will help you to focus on the things you want instead of the things you don't.

3. **Personal:** Your soul goals are personal to you. They're something you can have direct control over. As much as we would all love to change other people's behaviours and actions sometimes, your soul goals are about what *you* are creating, and why it matters in the wholeness of your life.

4. **Possible:** While your soul goals should stretch you and feel both exciting and a little scary, which is completely normal, they must be within the realms of what's achievable. You can't make winning the lottery an inevitability, but you do have power over things you can bring into being with your vision, intention and actions.

5. **Powerful:** Your soul goals should give you the full tingles. They are aligned to your values, and make you want to jump out of bed each morning. If they don't give you the feels, then they are not for you!

This is an example of using the five Ps to create BIG, BOLD, BEAUTIFUL goals with soul. I've marked up below where each of the five Ps comes into play …

"It's February, this time next year. I have created an opportunity (P1), within my current role at work, to develop a mentoring programme for my team. This has enabled me to secure a healthy training budget for a course that I have found to be super-inspiring (P2). I completed the course in September, and I have been able to bring my learnings into my own mindset of growth, confidence and creativity within my job role, and influence the wider team. I feel full of inspiration; I love making a positive difference to my team, and progressing my career (P3). It has been challenging, but all the hours of training were worth it (P4). Those around me comment on how beneficial the work is (P5). I am engaged, motivated and excited to do more, so that I can make a wider contribution, both to the business and my career."

Imagine your soul goals like writing a story of your BIG, BOLD, BEAUTIFUL life, and bringing it into existence, simply by crafting the storyline and plot. Being in alignment with your own life's story means you can co-create using your vision, values, dreams and desires. Unleash your wild imagination for a life that feels BIG, BOLD and BEAUTIFUL in every way.

Get ready to write your best-selling story of a lifetime and bring it into BIG, BOLD, BEAUTIFUL being by creating an Expansive Vision Map that brings your soul goals to life.

Are you ready? Let's GO!

YOUR EXPANSIVE VISION MAP

Now that you've explored the elements of what make up BIG, BOLD, BEAUTIFUL goals with soul, through the 5Ps of powerful goal setting, it's time to bring them to the party to create a vision map that provides a full and visceral experience of your energy, goals and intentions. A vision map is where you get to plug the destination into the sat nav, and create the map that's going to get you where you want to be. You take all of your soul goals and create a 360 view of what your BIG, BOLD, BEAUTIFUL life gets to be. It's the opportunity for you to dream big, and anchor what you truly desire in one beautiful and inspiring place.

It doesn't matter when you decide to create a vision map – you can do one at the beginning of the year, your birthday, the beginning of Spring, or simply any time you're looking to freshen up the vibe for your BIG, BOLD, BEAUTIFUL life.

Creating a BIG, BOLD, BEAUTIFUL vision map is the perfect opportunity to pause and take stock.

The power of looking at all areas of your life by creating a BIG, BOLD, BEAUTIFUL vision map is that, by looking at the 360 view of everything that's important to you, you can see how each area of your life supports the others. It highlights how you can create expansion in all areas, rather than focusing solely on one, at the detriment of something else.

Think of it like this … say you have a side hustle where you focus on empowering and supporting people – what I would call a heart-centred business – and you've been working on it for a couple of years. Up until now it's been ticking over, but it's not really bringing you the kind of income that means you can leave your salaried job. You decide at the beginning of the year to really go for it. It's time to make this side hustle a full-time thing. You know the work is important, and that you can reach many more people than you do right now. The income from your business will help you do that. Your values are freedom and adventure, so you need to make sure you are not working all hours; you need time to enjoy life. The opportunities and income you generate will allow you to do the things you love.

Great. But.

If you're not considering all aspects, and just focus on growing your side hustle, that hustle sees you working day and night until you barely have time for anything else in your life. By the end of the year you've reached your financial targets, but you are burnt out. Your clients are more demanding than they've ever been. You aren't enjoying the work any more, and you wonder if you can really keep going at the pace you have been, just to keep the money coming in.

Phew! Sounds exhausting and not sustainable in any way. And I don't want that for you and your life. It's not BIG, it's not BOLD and it certainly isn't BEAUTIFUL.

What if you could create expansion in all areas of your life instead of focusing so hard on one thing that everything else suffers? In this scenario, what if you could create expansion in your revenue and business, as well as creating precious time with your family and your partner? What if there was time for things that helped you to feel good and nourished your soul to give you energy and motivation for your work?

So, let's dive in to creating your expansive vision map to create your BIG, BOLD, BEAUTIFUL life by using those juicy soul goals that are bursting with excitement to get going.

A quick note – you don't need to worry about the "how" yet; this is about creating from a place of curiosity and expansion. You will explore how you start making these things happen as we get going on taking action in STEP TWO.

EXERCISE

CREATE YOUR BIG, BOLD, BEAUTIFUL VISION MAP

Your BIG, BOLD, BEAUTIFUL Vision Map is based on a simple but powerful coaching tool called the Wheel of Life. The "wheel" or vision map will help you discover areas of significance in your life, along with where you are right now in relation to those areas, and then where you would like to be within a specific timeframe. I love using the vision map at the beginning of any 12-month cycle, but you can choose any timeframe you wish. The shorter the timeframe, the more specific you need to get!

This exercise comes in three parts:

- Part One is about discovering the significant areas of your life.
- Part Two is about calibrating to see where you are right now in each of these priority areas.
- Part Three is about applying your BIG, BOLD, BEAUTIFUL soul goals in each of your priority areas.

To create your vision map you will need a large piece of paper, or you can create sections in your journal. To begin, draw a large circle that takes up most of the page, and a small circle in the centre of the large one. Then, draw equal lines through both circles that segment them into eight equal parts (like cutting a pizza into slices).

In the smaller circle mark 10 points along the centre line, with 0 in the centre, finishing with 10 at the outer edge of the smaller circle.

Here's what it will look like:

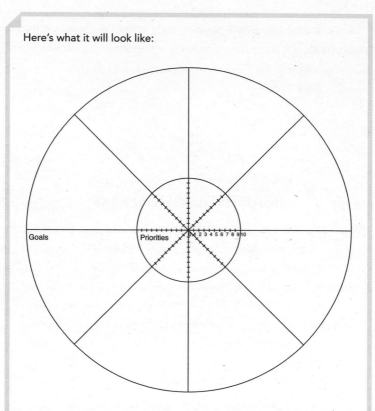

Goals · Priorities · 0 1 2 3 4 5 6 7 8 9 10

Part One: Define your key priority areas.

To begin, you are going to explore the eight key priority areas of your life. These are the things that are most important to you and make up the 360 of your life. They are likely to be along the same lines as the values you identified earlier. They could include things such as work, business, purpose, family, love, money, socializing, wellbeing, creativity, adventure, health, spirituality, finances, home life. If you get stuck, revisit your values (p. 16) and ask yourself what's so important that if it weren't in your life, it would cause things to be lacking, difficult or empty.

Write one key priority area in each of the segments of the smaller circle.

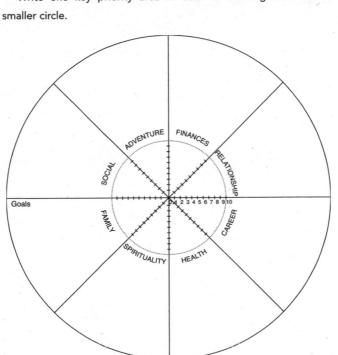

Part Two: Calibrate where you are right now.

Score where you feel your life is in relation to each of these priority areas. Give each segment a score of 0-10, where 0 is that it's nowhere near where you want it to be, and 10 is everything is exactly as you wish it to be. Mark a line across the segment relating to the score you give each priority area. Don't overthink it or judge what you are scoring; this is simply to get an overview of where you are and where you can create expansion.

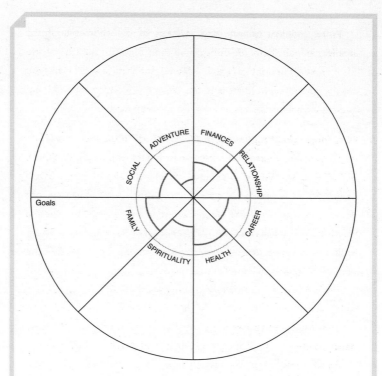

Once you've scored where you feel you are right now, take a look at your wheel. Is there anything that surprises you? Are there any areas where you scored higher, or lower, than you expected? What are the areas of your wheel that you scored higher on that you would like to keep where they are? Which are the areas that you didn't realize would be quite as low as they are?

If this were the wheel you were putting on your car to take you on a journey to your BIG, BOLD, BEAUTIFUL life, how easy would the ride be? Would it be a little bumpy? Would it take a long time because your wheel is so small?

Take a moment to write down your reflections. It's important to simply observe where you are starting out from, with the knowledge of where you are right now, rather than getting caught up in why you are not where you want them to be. We get to work on shifting them and creating expansion in all areas on the map next.

Part Three: Creating your BIG, BOLD, BEAUTIFUL soul goals.
It's time to take yourself on a creative love date with your BIG, BOLD, BEAUTIFUL life. Fill up the outer wheel with all your BIG, BOLD BEAUTIFUL soul goals for each priority area, but before you get going ... and this is not to be missed: date the top of your wheel a year from today, or whatever date you decide you would like to have brought your goals into being by. If it's six months from now, put the date at the top as six months from today.

This is because you are going to write your BIG, BOLD, BEAUTIFUL soul goals on your vision map as if it is the date you've written at the top of the map. You are sharing what has come into being in all those delicious priority areas of your BIG, BOLD, BEAUTIFUL life.

If you love writing long-form, you can go to town and write the story of your BIG, BOLD, BEAUTIFUL life a year from now. Or, if you prefer that your goals are succinct and more measurable, you can keep focused by creating three simple soul goals per segment. The key is to make sure they are as **specific** and **motivating** as possible so that your brain, mind and body know what's going down. Whatever goals you are putting down should have you fizzing with excitement.

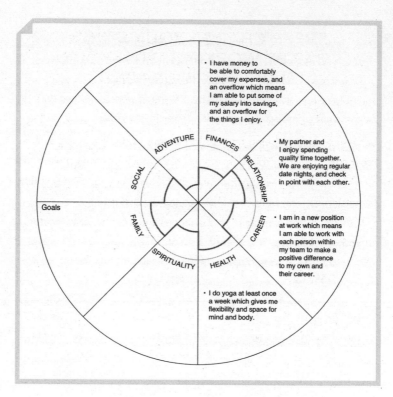

Once you have completed your vision map, you can either keep it somewhere safe to reference as you start working on getting focused and taking action in STEP TWO, or you can keep it somewhere safe you can come back to on the date you've written on the top of the map. I think you're going to be pretty amazed at what you notice when you come back to it!

When I've worked with clients on creating their vision map, I always tell them to be open and curious about what comes next, and to watch out for miracles! You will be amazed at how quickly some of what you've written down starts coming into being – sometimes, in the most unexpected ways. If you find yourself saying "Well, that's weird ..." it's not! The wheels are literally in motion, and it's time to jump on board.

SUPER-CHARGE YOUR VISION MAP BY WORKING WITH YOUR SUBCONSCIOUS MIND

The subconscious mind is a powerful force. It makes up around 95% of our brain and body power, and programmes how we think, feel and behave. As well as being responsible for our bodily functions, such as breathing, digesting, blinking – and pretty much everything we don't have to think about – it is responsible for creating our day-to-day reality, by making happen what our conscious mind wants it to do.

I think of the conscious and subconscious mind like a powerful computer processor. The conscious mind is the input, which provides instructions to the subconscious mind. Your vision map is the perfect example of this. Once the vision map has helped you to plan what you want to make happen, your subconscious provides a set of data and instructions to make it happen.

To put more power behind what you are creating, read through your vision map before you go to bed. Your subconscious mind is going to start filtering and sorting the information you are giving it, your brain will start firing up its synapses, and your body and brain are going to prepare to make your BIG, BOLD, BEAUTIFUL life happen. As well as this you can turbo-charge your vision map and soul goals by:

✓ Speaking them out loud.
✓ Visualizing them happening.
✓ Talking about them as if they're already happening. (They are.)
✓ Exercising them into being – I love swimming, running or lifting weights to bring body and mind power together. Think about your vision as you are carrying out these forms of exercise …
  • Swimming, for flow
  • Running, for going the distance
  • Weights, for strength and determination

You can learn more about activating your subconscious mind through your dreams in the Dream Casting Breakout ritual at the end of this step.

ENERGETICALLY IMPRINTING YOUR FUTURE IN THE NOW

Now that you've started to communicate to yourself and your conscious mind what you are creating and what you are bringing into clear vision with your BIG, BOLD, BEAUTIFUL life, you are going to super-charge it by taking it into every fibre of your being by creating an energetic and embodied imprint. This is where you bring all parts of you into alignment; mind, body, soul and all of your juicy energy, so you're left in no doubt that this thing is happening!

Everything that you are creating with right now is energy – the people, the money, the opportunities, the creativity, the collaborations ... all of it! As you bring them into existence, you activate the energy to vibrate at the frequency that they match with.

And you're off to an incredible start, because getting your BIG, BOLD, BEAUTIFUL soul goals written down is already 50% of the way there. Now, you're going to dial it up to 80-90% by creating energetic connections through a process called "sensory anchoring".

WHAT IS SENSORY ANCHORING?

As the brain doesn't know the difference between real and imagined, when you "anchor" an embodied, felt, sensory experience, you are connecting to what you've created on your vision map – the body feels it as if it's already here, your brain creates the neural pathways in accordance to it already being here, and the energy rises to meet it.

WHAT IS A SENSORY, EMBODIED EXPERIENCE?

A sensory, embodied experience is one where everything comes online – all your senses are lit, your senses come alive – what you hear (auditory), what you feel (kinaesthetic), what you see (visual), what you can smell (olfactory) and even what you can taste (gustatory) are all activated within your brain, your central nervous system, your mind and your body.

Love the sound of this? Want to play? The next and last exercise in this step will have you rocking your BIG, BOLD BEAUTIFUL life like it's one big party!

EXERCISE

CREATE AN EMBODIED SENSORY EXPERIENCE

Get your sparkles and get ready to dazzle as you step into an embodied sensory experience for what you've created on your vision map, with this creative visualization exercise.

Make sure you are somewhere you can sit or lie down undisturbed for around 10–15 minutes. Close your eyes, or soften your gaze.

Bring awareness to your breath with some deep refreshing inhales and exhales.

Continue to breathe deeply as you become aware of the chair or bed holding you. Know that wherever you are sitting or lying down, you are being supported as you go on this sensory adventure.

In your mind's eye imagine that you are at a New Year's Eve party. It's the kind of party or gathering that you most love to attend. The guests are the people you love spending time with the most.

Notice where this party is, and who's there.

What is the venue? The room you're in? Take a look around at what you can see around you. Take in the detail. What are you sitting on? What sounds can you hear? Do you have a drink in your hand? Maybe there's food. Take a sip or a bite. It's your favourite.

Take a look down at what you are wearing. It's the kind of outfit that makes you feel great. Feel the fabric on your skin, notice the patterns or colour of what you've got on. Those you've seen already this evening have complimented you on how great you look, and you feel it. Your hair is great, your skin is glowing ... You are glowing.

Notice who you're in conversation with. Maybe you're talking to someone you love to talk to. They love hearing what you've been doing. Maybe you are talking to a few close friends. Whoever it is, you see them beaming at you as you share what you've been doing and creating in the year that's just been.

As you share more about what you've been doing, and what you've achieved, you can feel your soul lighting up from the inside out. You are proud of what you've done. You are content and fulfilled. You can feel the fizz of excitement among your friends as you share with them more of what's to come in the next year. You can feel the electricity and the buzz of energy and love that comes from your connection with them and you. Their eyes light up as they see you in your flow.

As the clock strikes midnight, you raise a toast to the year that's been, and feel gratitude for everything in it. You are alive and excited about the expansion ahead of you, eager for the next 12 months to come. Anything feels possible.

Take some deep breaths as you bask in the glow of this BIG, BOLD, BEAUTIFUL embodied experience you've just created. Notice where you feel it in your body.

Gently open your eyes. Give yourself a moment of gratitude for going on this epic adventure.

Journal about anything that came up in your embodied sensory visualization then write down how it deepened the connection to your BIG, BOLD, BEAUTIFUL vision map.

Now, as you explore deeper into the next steps, bring your soul goals and your vision map, because it's time to bring them into BIG, BOLD, BEAUTIFUL being.

STEP ONE REVIEW TIME

Let's take a moment of pause and reflection as you deep dive into the first step of your BIG, BOLD, BEAUTIFUL life – CREATE THE VISION. Here are your check-in points for what you have explored in STEP ONE. You have:

✓ Connected to the *power of intention* by creating the energetic alignment between you and the BIG, BOLD, BEAUTIFUL life you are creating.

✓ Got clear on what you are saying "goodbye" and "hello" to in your BIG, BOLD, BEAUTIFUL life by carrying out an e*nergetic stock check.*

✓ Connected to *your core values* by carrying out a value elicitation exercise that will become the inner compass to guide you on your BIG, BOLD BEAUTIFUL vision quest.

✓ Learned about *"move away from" and "move toward" goals* by flipping the script to connect to the expansive, motivating things you want for your BIG, BOLD, BEAUTIFUL life.

✓ Set the destination in the sat nav for your BIG, BOLD, BEAUTIFUL life by creating *soul goals.*

✓ Explored the 360 view of your life to create expansion in all areas by learning how to create a *BIG, BOLD, BEAUTIFUL Vision Map.*

✓ Energetically imprinted your BIG, BOLD, BEAUTIFUL soul goals into the present moment through an *embodied sensory experience* visualization.

Now that you've created your vision map and your embodied BIG, BOLD, BEAUTIFUL goals with soul, it's time to move on to STEP TWO, the one where you make sure the shiny squirrels don't throw you off-course!

But before you do, here's the first of your BIG, BOLD, BEAUTIFUL Breakout Rituals. Why not try a spot of dream-casting for some soulful energy activation that will power up your BIG, BOLD, BEAUTIFUL vision while you sleep and consolidate everything you've learned so far.

BREAKOUT RITUAL
SLEEP RITUAL & DREAM-CASTING

This sleep ritual is the perfect way to put more power behind your BIG, BOLD, BEAUTIFUL vision by activating the power of your subconscious mind through dreaming.

Dreams occur at the rapid eye movement (REM) stage of sleep, the first of which generally occurs around an hour to an hour and a half after you fall asleep. It's when you have your most vivid dreams, whether you're aware of them or not. Dreaming is when the subconscious mind is filtering and processing everything you've input through the conscious mind in the last 24–48 hours. You consciously created the vision map. Now, you can activate the subconscious through your dreaming state to fuel your BIG, BOLD, BEAUTIFUL vision into reality.

The subconscious mind works with symbols, shapes, archetypes and through storytelling. This is why dreams don't often seem to make sense to our rational, thinking mind. But through the language of the subconscious mind, dreams can offer insights into what's going on.

You will activate both the potential of your vision map, and the power of your subconscious mind through dream state, in this ritual.

1. *Create your sleep ritual*
   - As with all rituals, prepare yourself and your space for a ritual to take place.
   - Have a bath, switch off your devices, make sure you're nice and warm and ready for sleep.
   - You can prepare the space in which you are sleeping by making it as comfortable as possible. Have fresh sheets, soften the lights.
   - Have a journal and pen near where you sleep so you can access it on waking.

- Have your vision map close by. You may want to read it through before you set your intentions, or have it in an envelope.
- Spray an air or pillow spritz with either moon water (water which has been charged by the new or full moon), or any kind of spritz that will relax you (lavender or rose is perfect).
- If you have an amethyst crystal (the dreaming crystal), have this close to where you are sleeping. You could also use it to charge the moon water ahead of time.
- Light a candle.
- Climb into bed and get ready for sleep.

2. *Create your intention*
   - Breathe deeply and ask your dreams to activate your vision map to provide you with some kind of guidance, ideas or messages that might be useful to you.
   - You may want to journal some prompts or questions on what it is exactly that you would like to know from your dreams – any guidance, ideas, or messages, a specific action or idea.
   - State an intention in your heart and mind that you will remember and learn from your dreams. (You don't have to do anything here; just make the invitation to open your heart and mind.)

3. *Let the dreams commence*
   - Soften your gaze as you look into the flame of the candle, inviting you to be lulled into a restful sleep.
   - Again, you don't have to do anything here, other than letting yourself fall into a deep sleep, and your dreams will do their work.

4. *On waking*
   - There's a sweet spot of time between coming out of sleep and being consciously aware, called the Hypnopompic

State. It's when you are becoming awake, but are not yet fully awake. It's often when the subconscious is bringing its messages to you in a way that starts to make sense, or can create hallucinations (such as you think you're awake, but random things seem to be happening).

- Whatever comes through from the messages in this state or through your dreams (by way of a clear message, symbols, people or stories) it is all information that can be extremely useful to you.
- Sometimes, the answer presents itself clearly on the cusp of the awakened state.
- Have your journal to hand, so that you can capture any clear messages, or make note of your thoughts or dreams as you wake up.
- Don't try to analyse anything that doesn't make sense straight away; just write anything and everything that comes up as you wake up.

5. *Throughout the day (and beyond)*
   - You may come back to your journal throughout the day to check in on what your dreams have gifted you in relation to your vision map.
   - Become curious about any signs, symbols, words, messages, people or animals that your dreams brought you; they may hold clues.
   - This might show up as people getting in contact, or something else happening in your day.
   - It might take a few days for things to become clear.
   - Be patient, be open, be curious as to what comes up. The gifts your dreams give you may be hiding in plain sight in your everyday life. Your job is to pay attention.

This exercise will take practice, so come back to it on a regular basis when you are reconnecting to your vision map and soul goals.

STEP TWO

FIND YOUR FOCUS

So, you've created your vision map, and you have your soul goals, now it's time to explore how you are going to bring your vision, intention and soul goals into fruition … making your BIG, BOLD, BEAUTIFUL life a reality, while – and most importantly – making sure you don't get side-tracked at every turn!

You've started on the road to creating that BIG, BOLD and BEAUTIFUL vision for what's ahead. How freaking exciting. But oh, wait … What's that over there? Squirrel!

What I know to be true from doing this work over the past 15-plus years is that you can create those BIG, BOLD, BEAUTIFUL soul goals and they will stay on the vision board of dreams forever. You can sit in your manifestation pants all day willing and waiting for the good stuff to come your way … but unless you are blending intention with action, to start bringing those goals into focus, then they will stay a blur of hope and dreams on your vision board.

While 70% of the work has been done through the creation of your BIG, BOLD, BEAUTIFUL soul goals, it's now all about the other 30%. It's time to bring those goals to life, and crucially, not get side-tracked or stray so far off the path that you forget where you wanted to be in the first place (which is all too easy to do, believe me). This is about creating a powerful blend of commitment, action and awareness as you move forward on your BIG, BOLD, BEAUTIFUL path.

TAKING ACTION WITHOUT THE ANGUISH

In your BIG, BOLD, BEAUTIFUL LIFE taking action doesn't have to mean extra hustle. Yes, it does mean changing behaviours and working toward your soul goals, but it doesn't mean flinging yourself around at such a high speed you end up burning out because you can't keep the momentum going – even if you are feeling the full power of motivation right now. And it doesn't mean doing ALL. THE. THINGS. Because that only leads to a spaghetti junction of overwhelm and over-complication. Very quickly, what you have envisioned on your vision map feels all too much, and what started with a beautifully simple idea becomes an unwieldy beast that you just want to run away and hide from. And then there's the squirrels, the glossy, shiny squirrels, those tricky little attention grabbers that seem to appear out of nowhere and want to lead you Pied Piper style away from where you want to be.

It doesn't feel BIG, BOLD, or remotely BEAUTIFUL, so why does it happen? Well, this is where the sneaky fear and ego will come on in and try to over-complicate things in a trickster way to keep you from failing on the thing you really want. Your subconscious is scared you're going to fail so it puts things in the way to make sure you do … Yes, it's a mind-flip, but once you're aware you can check in to make sure you're not knocked off the path.

We will explore this – and more – in this step, so you can keep your eyes on the prize and stay focused on your BIG, BOLD, BEAUTIFUL vision, while creating momentum each and every day by breaking everything down into simple actions and taking a step-by-step approach.

Focus, clarity and momentum are the ultimate power trio when it comes to making your vision a reality. They will be the number one things to help you get crystal clear on what you need to do, how you need to do it, and what conditions and support you will need to make it happen.

TRIED AND TESTED

Everything I am sharing with you is tried and tested and is an evolving process. On a personal level, I have been able to get out of my own way by unpicking and unlearning patterns of behaviour. I'm aware of my narratives of over-working and burning out. I have an awareness of my underlying need to prove something to ... well, goodness knows who ... all mixed together with an (un)healthy dose of how society views what it is to lead a "successful" life. It's a lot to unpack, but it gets to be the ultimate act of rebellion – to take what seems over-complicated, and come back to a place of simplicity. When you tune back in to your core values, get clear on your desires and filter out the noise, you gain the focus to bring the BIG, BOLD and BEAUTIFUL into existence.

Some of this, or all of this, will be going on for you too. Some of it you might be aware of, and some of it is running an unconscious dialogue, but it is going to be different. You do get to step off the grind of overwhelm.

This section will enable you to:

- Bring your BIG visions to life; by keeping an eye on the bigger picture and lifting yourself up and out of the detail you're able to focus on what you ultimately want to achieve, rather than what you haven't yet done.
- Be BOLD with the actions you take, no matter how big or small those actions are. You can focus on taking the truest action for you. That's instead of doing the things you think you should be doing for fear of getting it wrong, or worrying about what people will think of you. You can concentrate on your vision and be guided by your values, because they are yours and yours alone.

- Bring your BEAUTIFUL life into being on your own terms, with much more presence to enjoy the rich experience of what you are creating by being in tune with your creative energy and passion.

IN STEP TWO YOU WILL:

✓ Explore why and where *you're over-complicating it* and how you can shift out of overwhelm, into opportunity, to ensure you keep on the path toward your BIG, BOLD, BEAUTIFUL soul goals.

✓ Learn how to recognize and *ditch the distractions* to make sure you're not taking your eyes off the BIG, BOLD, BEAUTIFUL vision you have set out for yourself. And how you can turn distraction into simple micro-actions that lift your soul goals from paper and into reality.

✓ Unlock the *power of the one-degree shift* to create a tidal wave of change-taking steps that focus on ONE thing at a time as you take aligned action on your soul goals ... and how to bring celebration into each action to create powerful energy and momentum.

✓ Understand how *productivity is the love child of focus,* and how working with your energy is the juice to get it flowing. You will close down some of the million tabs you have open on your brain, stop procrastinating, and feel good about taking aligned action from a place of being in flow with your rhythms.

Get ready to roll up your beautiful sleeves and don your love specs as we bring things into BIG, BOLD, BEAUTIFUL focus. It's time to get this disco ball show on the road and start creating some serious movement and momentum toward your BIG, BOLD, BEAUTIFUL soul goals!

We are freaking doing it!

DEALING WITH DISTRACTIONS

When I started off on the path of working in alignment with purpose, and especially when I stepped into building my coaching business, I would get excited by a million ideas before lunchtime. Sometimes, I would get excited by a million ideas before I had even gotten out of the shower. I still do! I blame it on being born on a new moon. I love creating new things. I love seeking out new opportunities. And most of all, I love this work, with all of my heart.

The challenge is that I would try and action them all in one go, my heart skipping like an excited puppy, but my mind a tumbled mess of what to do first. I would start lots of things, and have all the tabs open on my brain, which made it impossible to complete anything or see any of them through. Or, because I was so excited about the direction of travel and the unlimited possibilities of what I could do, I would agree to pretty much everything that would come my way, without really figuring out if it was the best or truest direction of travel toward my ultimate BIG, BOLD, BEAUTIFUL destination. Yes, it felt exciting, and yes it felt exhilarating, but I ended up sand blasting a lot of different things in an incredibly scatter-gun approach, without having any clear strategy in place. And because I was still working on being the ultimate people-pleaser I would end up being super-busy, overwhelmed, resentful and on my knees!

Can you relate?

There is a natural excitement to it all. You will get excited about your soul goals or a new idea you channel. You will want it here, and you will want it NOW. The ideas might explode out of you like a glitter cannon of possibility. That might be happening with you right now. Following STEP ONE you might be alive with a million ideas and endless opportunities.

I call this the "and thens". You start with a simple, beautiful idea and then add something else to it, and then something else, and then something else and then something else ... until that beautifully simple idea becomes unrecognizable and seemingly impossible to achieve.

It's a sneaky form of self-sabotage. So, what can be done about it?

COULD YOU BE UPPER LIMITING YOURSELF?

This counterproductive behaviour is what Gay Hendricks, in his book *The Big Leap*, calls "creating an upper limit problem". He means that you divert attention away from making something great happen, and limit yourself and your potential, because ultimately, you're afraid you're going to fail or fuck it up.

For example, you go all out on a project at work. It's something that is really important to you and will put you in line for a positive review, a potential promotion and a pay rise. But you do something at the last minute, which leaves you feeling unprepared and lacking the confidence to deliver, so you fall short on delivering and miss out on a promotion.

This is when you take a perfectly simple idea and then the ego steps in to question everything about it. *Surely it can't be that simple ... Someone else must be doing this ... Surely this should be more challenging than it is ... Surely to do something that has weight and meaning, it is supposed to feel like hard work ...* Much of this comes from outdated patterns and programmes, telling you that things have to be hard to deserve the reward, or that the simplest action is the lazy option.

We give ourselves many, many sticks to beat ourselves with! When you accept that you can put the stick down, things become a lot more simple, and enjoyable. You can get out of your own way and into flow. You can give yourself the time, space and energy you need, and create a test, learn, adapt approach to taking things step by step.

EXERCISE

EXPLORE YOUR LIMITING TENDENCIES

Explore your over-complicating tendencies with some of these exploratory questions, so you can gain awareness of where they might be stopping you, before you start.

I know I start over-complicating things when ...
Example: "I take a simple idea and add loads of other things to it to make it much bigger than when I started out."

....

....

....

I self-sabotage by ...
Example: "Not giving myself enough time to complete things," or "I will do everything else other than the thing I really want."

....

....

....

My "upper limit" tendencies have shown up in the past as ...
Example: "Putting so much detail into an assignment that I know it's going to be near-impossible to deliver." or "Saying yes to something, knowing I had way too much on my plate meant I didn't give the thing that was most important the care and attention it needed, so I wasn't happy with either outcome."

....

....

....

Come back to these questions as you explore navigating your BIG, BOLD, BEAUTIFUL life and creating even BIGGER, BOLDER and more BEAUTIFUL goals. Believe me when I say that uncovering your patterns is not a one-time-only experience, and there's always more to peel away and discover about what you unconsciously and sometimes consciously do, to get in your own way!

DITCHING THE DISTRACTIONS

So, you've identified your goals in STEP ONE. And now, you know what's likely to knock you off-course. How many times have you found yourself getting revved up with excitement to start making that BIG, BOLD, BEAUTIFUL thing happen, only to find yourself getting side-tracked by something other than what you want to be doing? You tell yourself that today is going to be the day. You wake up full of energy and ideas, only to find yourself a few hours later, having done every damn thing other than what you had planned to do that day. Maybe you tell yourself, "That's OK, tomorrow is another day, I'll get started then," only to find yourself the next day having gone off on a complete tangent from the thing you were going to get started on.*

*I'm chuckling to myself as I write this, because I went online to find a reference relevant to this topic, only to go down a scroll hole for 15 minutes and completely forgetting what I went to my browser for!

Another day comes along, you get invited out for coffee, and you're out of the door before you've even finished the thought of, "Oh, why not? I can start this tomorrow." And let's not even get started on the household chores you can find to do if you're working from home. Some of us have never had a cleaner oven!

PROCRASTINATION PARTY

If you find yourself getting side-tracked by procrastination, and pretty much everything other than what you want to be working on, then you know that the shiny, shiny squirrels are having a procrastination party and your name is well and truly on the list!

Procrastination when it comes to doing something new, daunting, exciting, and which has true value and importance to you, is a completely natural thing. Most people are prone to procrastination. We all have different styles of working at things – some of us are last-minute crammers, and some of us put things off until it's absolute crunch time, because we find we work better under pressure. It's important to note that if you have ADD, dyslexia or ADHD, executive functioning issues may well interfere with how you get things done.

The truth is that procrastination is entirely normal, but if you find that it's going on for too long, and that you continue to procrastinate despite knowing you are likely to be worse off for not having worked toward your BIG, BOLD, BEAUTIFUL soul goals, then there could be other things at play.

So, if deep down we know that ongoing procrastination may not be serving us, why do we do it?

Procrastination for protection

Generally, procrastination is an in-built safety mechanism that protects us from things our ego feels is beyond its levels of comfort. It serves as the ultimate avoidance tactic, so when we find something … anything …

to do other than the thing we had planned to do, it gives temporary respite for the fear critters playing up within us.

Of course, when you're on the nowhere train at Procrastination Station it could well be down to self-belief, and how confident you feel about your ability to get the thing done. We will explore how you can work with your self-beliefs, and build your self-empowerment toolkit to deal with a crisis of confidence, in STEPS THREE and FIVE.

Procrastination as a reward

Sometimes, procrastination is a double bind of relief and reward, which provides instant gratification by providing a hit of the feel-good dopamine chemical in the brain. Doing smaller, seemingly achievable non-contributing actions such as organizing your sock drawer, is instantly rewarding. Whereas the rewards for the actions that might take more time, thought and effort, appear too far in the distance. Instant reward may only be a double-tap or a scroll away, but it leaves your BIG, BOLD, BEAUTIFUL life further out of reach.

Right now it's time to take that BIG, BOLD, BEAUTIFUL vision board off the wall and start bringing it into aligned action. But before you go off to clean that spot behind the sofa that has never seen the light of day, come with me, because we're going to explore some tools to help you create focus and take action.

TOOLS TO MOVE BEYOND PROCRASTINATION
Choose your focus

Before we go any further, grab your vision map from STEP ONE (p. 27) and look at the area of focus you want to start working with. Don't necessarily go for what you think is going to be the easiest, but rather what's going to create the kind of BIG, BOLD, BEAUTIFUL impact you came here to explore in the first place.

And then breathe! Because what you are looking at in front of you may be 6 months or 12 months out from here. So, if it feels too daunting in this very moment, it's because you're racing ahead to the finish line, without having yet done any training or preparation, let alone having yet got off the starting line!

In this very moment the first place to start is to decide what area you are going to focus on, and then chunk that down into achievable and realistic milestones. Once you have decided which segment on your vision map you are going to work with, you can delve into creating actionable steps.

The Micro-Actions and the One Degree Shift

As you will no doubt recognize in yourself, procrastination and distraction happen when things feel too big to handle, and even though focusing on the area that you are going to take action on first is a great step forward, that alone doesn't mean that your motivation and productivity levels are going to kick you into gear.

Don't get me wrong – it's an incredible step forward to distill it down to one area of focus when you consider all that powerful vision that was living inside of you can now see the light of day – but it's the only way you are going to get on the ladder that will help you climb each step. So, you get to explore each step within that one segment, and chunk them down into manageable mini steps – micro-actions.

This is where you get to take a dive into the reality of all of the bits that make up the whole, and create tangible action and priority plans in the first area of the vision map you're working with. You'll break it down, break it down, break it down into bite-sized micro-actions that you can create a plan around, then start working that plan.

Think of micro-actions as one-degree shifts. What could happen toward making your BIG, BOLD, BEAUTIFUL dreams a reality if you took the smallest of shifts each and every day? And then what could happen if you took a one-degree shift each day over the course of the 12 months that you are planning on your BIG, BOLD, BEAUTIFUL vision map? Yep! You would be a full circle (and more) from where you're starting out from.

And, yes, you may have that voice in your head when you first look at your vision map telling you that it's never going to happen, or overwhelming you with the prospect of how you could ever make it so ... but if you keep coming back to micro-actions, each and every day over the course of 12 months ... well, that's where that powerful intention and action come together to have a magical love child and your BIG, BOLD, BEAUTIFUL life comes into the world.

BREAKING DOWN YOUR VISION TO MAKE IT A REALITY

So, let's start making that dream a reality. This is where I begin with every single one of my clients, following the vision map creation – by deciding which area is going to get that love-in action first. You know what you want, but how are you going to get there?

Work your way through these exercises and you'll find you're well on your way!

EXERCISE

SET MICRO-ACTIONS TO ACHIEVE YOUR GOALS

Choose the segment on your BIG, BOLD, BEAUTIFUL vision map that you will work with first. Think about what milestone you will have in place six months from now, which is halfway to achieving your 12-month BIG, BOLD, BEAUTIFUL vision in that segment area. If it helps you can take a look at the section on SMART goals (p. 21).

Working backwards from there, create a milestone for three months (90 days) from now, which demonstrates you are on that halfway marker point to your six-month milestone. Don't overwhelm yourself by making it too detailed at this point; keep your milestones clear and simple.

Below is an example of the 12-month goal, 6-month milestone and your first 90-day milestone.

SEGMENT AREA	WORK/BUSINESS
A 12-month soul goal	I am hosting a group weekend retreat for 10 women based around creativity and wellbeing in a beautiful location.
6-month milestone	I have the venue, date and location confirmed, so that I can start marketing the event.
First 3-month (90 day) milestone.	I have researched venues, got costs and availability. I have a rough date in the diary and have a costs spreadsheet. I have an idea of how much I will need to charge guests for the weekend.

OK, now it's your turn ... Take your area of focus over to your journal, or planner, and first:

- Identify the SEGMENT AREA
- Then the 12-month soul goal
- Your 6-month milestone
- Then your first 3-month (90 day) milestone.

Once you've got clear on these, take a moment to consider how you will feel as you hit the quarter-stage point toward your BIG, BOLD, BEAUTIFUL 12-month vision in this segment?

Example: I am buzzing with excitement. It's absolutely perfect. I am feeling motivated to start pulling everything together.

EXERCISE

WORK THAT 90-DAY GOAL

Now, let's get some focus back on your first 3-month – 90-days – goals and actions.

Take a look at the elements of your first 90-day goal and break that down into three x monthly (30-day) key actions. Ask yourself: How does this split into simple and possible actions over the next three months?

Example:

Focus for month 1: Research venues online and reach out to find out about availability and costs.

Focus for month 2: Work out all the associated costs for the weekend. Create a costs spreadsheet and work out a pricing structure for the guests.

Focus for month 3: Visit potential venues and make a decision about which one will work best.

Your turn:

Focus for month 1: ....

Focus for month 2: ....

Focus for month 3: ....

Looking at the things you've split into simple and doable areas of focus and action over the next three months, break those down into even smaller chunks – micro-actions – that are going to take you one step forward in week-by-week steps. Remember to note down how much time you'll give yourself to do each bit.

MONTH 1 FOCUS

RESEARCHING VENUES	MICRO-ACTIONS	TIME IT WILL TAKE
Week 1:	• Start desk research to look for venues online / ask people who've hosted before for recommendations.	3-4 hours (across 2 days)
Week 2:	• Shortlist and start contacting venues by email and telephone. • Ask about costs and availability around the approximate dates I've set aside for the retreat.	3-4 hours (across 2 days)
Week 3:	• Start a costs spreadsheet: plug in venue costs, catering and other costs per head. • Shortlist 3 preferred venues and arrange visits.	4-5 hours (across 3 days)
Week 4:	• Visit 3 venues. • Make a decision about which will be best. • Update the costs spreadsheet and confirm a pricing structure for guests. • Book and pay the deposit for the venue.	3-4 hours (across 5 days)

Go back to your journal or planner, and replicate the table exercise to find out how your micro-actions split down into weekly bite-sized chunks over the next three months.

You can get really granular and break down your micro-actions into even smaller actions on a daily basis within each week, but it's not necessary, unless the idea of that really gets you buzzed!

Of course, this all has to work around your existing commitments, so it's important to get really clear on how you can fit this in around what else you have going on, because, well … life! I find it useful to get a calendar or planner out and start plotting when I am going to put the micro-actions into play for the first month only. Then, I plan out the next months as things start to take shape. Things are always a movable feast, but from this starting point you can have a clear idea of focus and actions.

EXERCISE

IDENTIFY POTENTIAL ROADBLOCKS

Now, it's important to know what could stop you from taking action, and where you might need help and support with your micro-actions as you hit the road. So, reviewing the first month of micro-actions in advance, filter them through these questions:

What can you do on your own? Where might you need to get support and help with any of the micro-actions you've listed? When will you reach out to make it happen?

....

....

....

....

....

What else might you need in order to get started?

....

....

....

....

....

What might stop you from taking these first steps?

....

....

....

....

....

What will you do, or what support will you get, to make sure that doesn't happen?

....

....

....

....

....

How will you celebrate the fact that you've taken the first BIG, BOLD, BEAUTIFUL 30-day steps toward the rest of your BIG, BOLD, BEAUTIFUL life? *If you need help with how you might celebrate, you can go to the 20 ideas for everyday celebration* (p. 238).

Don't skip this bit because celebration is as important as taking the action in the first place.

You've done it! Congratulations! You are already on your way to making your BIG, BOLD, BEAUTIFUL vision a reality by getting some focus and clarity on your next steps, and forming a plan of action to get there. Now it's time to bring action and energy together to make sure all parts of you are in alignment to create true momentum.

PRODUCTIVITY IS THE LOVE CHILD OF FOCUS AND WORKING WITH YOUR ENERGY

What we've explored so far in STEP TWO is kind of a coaching 101, and for someone who comes from a background of project management within creative environments, this is the kind of stuff I get really excited about. Seeing something tangible being brought to life from a vision and a creative idea, is nothing short of a miracle, and not one to take for granted.

Without creating the plan and breaking things down into those manageable micro-actions, most people get as far as creating the vision of a BIG, BOLD, BEAUTIFUL life, and then they stall. And herein is the truth – manifestation and wishing alone just don't cut it. You've got to meet the energy of your vision by taking the action.

Breaking things down into those micro-actions and driving on the open road of your BIG, BOLD, BEAUTIFUL adventure each day is ideal, but not everything works in a structured and linear way in life. There will be times when even the most carefully executed project plan of dreams goes out of the window. That doesn't mean that unless you do the thing you had planned on the day you planned to do it, your BIG, BOLD, BEAUTIFUL vision is never going to happen.

There are going to be times when you are on it, firing with all cylinders. This is where you might focus on "doing" or "thinking" actions, such as researching, getting bids written, focusing on a financial or marketing plan.

There are going to be times when your vibe is high, so you use the time to get out meeting people and networking, or creating and engaging with communities both online and in-person.

There are going to be times when you're more reflective than active. You might find that you feel connected to something within you that wants to come out. This is where you might spend time doing some introspective work, such as getting creative, or writing.

And then there are going to be times when you need rest. On these days you will find it hard to do anything, other than snuggling down into a sofa, under a blanket.

It's all action!

Sometimes, you will feel this ebb and flow of energy throughout several weeks, and sometimes you're going to feel it within a single day. Sometimes, you have lots of energy, sometimes you don't feel like you have much in the tank. The ebb and flow of your energy and motivation is a completely natural thing. This is due to the fact that you are not a machine running on factory settings to get something done. Neither are you computer-programmed to create a result based on a set of code input into an operating system. You are an energetic, cyclical being who oscillates with seasons, cycles, hormones, biology and even the Moon.

What your productivity and energy levels are like will be entirely different to someone else's; only you can work out what is going to work for you. By observing your own energy patterns, you can work with them, rather than against them, and this will put a stop to you being hard on yourself when you don't have the energy and focus that you did last week. It means that you can shift your focus to doing something that is more suited to the energy you are aligned with in that moment.

We're going to go deep into working with your energy to dial it up in STEP FOUR. For now, here's an overview of some of the things you can start thinking about, to help you tap in to the infinite power source of your own different levels of productivity through understanding energy at play.

HARNESS YOUR BIOLOGICAL ENERGY RHYTHMS FOR EFFECTIVE PRODUCTIVITY

We have natural rhythms going on within our bodies that affect our energy on a daily basis. Understanding your internal body clocks, or biological energy rhythms, helps to get you in step with the metaphorical jump rope of your productivity and energy levels. There are going to be times for taking action, and times for resting; by connecting to how this works for you will help you create an alignment to your own energy levels.

Here are some of the cycles and phases that you can start working with to align your BIG, BOLD, BEAUTIFUL soul goals with focused productivity and motivation levels:

CIRCADIAN RHYTHMS

The circadian rhythm (or cycle) is a 24-hour sleep / wake cycle, which tells your body when to wake up, when to eat, when to sleep, and even when to go to the loo! It's directly related to the amount of light received through the optical nerves in your eyes, telling your body when it should naturally be awake and alert, or when to slow down and get ready for sleep.

Humans are a diurnal (non-nocturnal) species, which means we are generally active during the day and sleep at night. Although an internal circadian clock is around 24 hours, there will be variations to circadian rhythms, and differences in the speed of your own individual rhythms. Ever considered yourself a morning person or a night owl? If your circadian clock runs faster than 24 hours, you may have more energy in the morning. If your clock runs slower than 24 hours, you might find you have more energy in the evening.

Getting to know and understand your circadian rhythm means you can find ways to work in flow with your own 24-hour biological cycle.

Here's a brief overview of a generalized circadian 24-hour cycle. It demonstrates how you might align your natural energy levels to certain tasks. Please be aware, this may be different for you, and various factors will be at play, but understanding general ebbs and flows of energy is a great place to start for you to become aware of your own energy fluctuations.

6am to 8am is the natural waking time. Blood pressure and cortisol levels (the stress hormone) rise to get you up and out of bed. This is the time of day that sets the tone for the rest of your day. It's good for:

✓ Intention setting for the day ahead
✓ Journalling
✓ Activating breath work
✓ Stretching or exercise

10am to midday is your most mentally alert time of the day. Your body temperature rises and alertness levels increase. 11am is usually peak productivity. Good for:

✓ A task or two on your to-do list
✓ Admin
✓ Planning & strategic thinking

1pm to 4pm is the time when your body starts slowing down a little, although it can also be the best time for co-ordination and fast reactions. You may find that you hit an energy lull between 3-4pm, so you might feel sluggish and in need of a 20-minute rest, or you might find yourself heading for the biscuit jar to get a sugary fix. Good for:

✓ Working on creative projects
✓ Physical projects
✓ Activating breath work
✓ Taking a nap or going for a walk

5pm to 8pm is the time when there's generally a burst of activity. Blood pressure increases in the early evening, which can be great for a burst of productivity. Good for:

✓ Another couple of tasks on your to-do list
✓ Finishing up some emails
✓ Exercise

From 9pm onwards melatonin (the sleep hormone) starts to kick in to prepare you for sleep. You should try to not look at devices that emit bright light after this time as they will interrupt your natural melatonin production. Good for:

✓ Journalling
✓ Reading
✓ Having a bath / another self-care activity, such as gentle stretching or meditation

Another quick note on biological rhythms: your body will release adrenaline and cortisol into your body if you're still awake past midnight. This is because it thinks that you are awake because there's something wrong, and it needs to be kept hyper-vigilant in case you're under attack. This is where you might find yourself wired, but tired; you might struggle to get to sleep, or to have the kind of rest-repair quality sleep that your brain and your body needs.

Individual body clocks will change based on a number of factors, such as: life-stage (teenage years, pregnancy, menopause), chronic health conditions, executive functioning conditions (ADHD, ADD) stress factors, eyesight problems affecting the amount of light entering the optical nerves in the eyes, high or low blood pressure, melatonin disorders, vitamin D deficiency, caffeine, stress, alcohol, night shifts, long work hours, jet lag … and so much more.

Changes in the seasons, and how much daylight you receive, can shift your natural circadian cycle up or down by a couple of hours.

ULTRADIAN RHYTHMS

While your circadian cycle works across 24 hours, you also have mini biological rhythms within them, called ultradian rhythms. These mini cycles, or energy waves, regulate energy, mood and cognitive function. They affect your thoughts, behaviour and actions. The word "ultradian" means "many times a day".

Throughout the night you're unlikely to be aware of these mini rhythms as your body goes through its natural 90-minute REM cycles of rest and repair. But during the day you have several waves of ultradian rhythms, which means your energy will naturally rise, peak, fall and then flatten out around every 90-120 minutes. The idea is that you work in alignment with a biological ultradian "rest-activity" wave, so be active for 90 minutes and then rest for 20 minutes. That way you can work more efficiently with your natural biological energy flows.

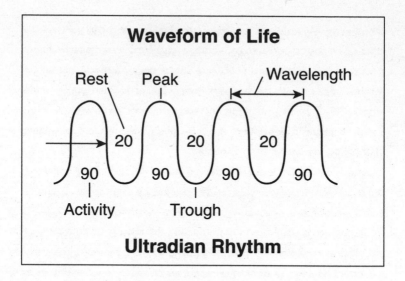

Here's how to get the most out of working on your BIG, BOLD, BEAUTIFUL soul goals in alignment with your ultradian rhythms, to help you stay on task and focused:

- Take one of your micro-actions (p. 52) and break it down into 60–90-minute chunks. Take the first chunk of activity and then work on it for that amount of time. If it's something that takes a lot of thinking or creative focus, notice when your energy starts to flag, or your concentration starts wandering. This is a cue that you're hitting the lowest point of an ultradian rhythm wave and you need to take a break.
- Use the 30-minute Pomodoro technique. This is a time management method, where you have 25 minutes of focus and 5 minutes of rest. It helps to break up a 90-minute ultradian rhythm cycle. You can set a timer for 25 minutes, to work on one of your micro-actions, and then stop for a break when the alarm goes off.

- Or, you could take a "brain break" of between 20–30 minutes, every 60–90 minutes. You could go for a walk, take a nap, meditate – the idea is that you are switching your brain off from the task you are working on. Scrolling doesn't count here!

Other ways to work with your ultradian rhythms throughout the day include:

- Practice Yoga Nidra, which is otherwise known as yogic sleep. Practising this deep relaxation practice for 30 minutes is said to be worth as much as three hours of deep restorative sleep.
- Have a dance break! If you've been sitting still for a long time then get some tunes on and move your body.
- Stop and sit! If you've been on the go for a long time then stop what you've been doing and have a rest for 15–20 minutes. Preferably, go outside so you can catch some vitamin D.
- Get creative. If you've been working on something that has taken up a lot of thinking space, get doodling or drawing as this will naturally turn your brain from doing to being, and will activate your parasympathetic (rest and digest) nervous system. I love taking a break to draw mandalas.
- Talk with a friend. Taking 20 minutes away from what you've been doing will switch the focus away from what you've been working on. That'll give your brain and body the rest it needs, before you go back to your next task.

THE SEASONS OF THE MENSTRUAL CYCLE:

There's a huge amount of BIG, BOLD, BEAUTIFUL wisdom in a menstrual cycle, if you have one. Even if you don't you can work with the power of your cyclical seasons, which you have within every 28-day cycle. (Skip to p. 69).

There are four key seasons or phases within any menstrual cycle, which are based on a 27 – 30 day cycle. Working with these phases within a menstrual cycle, by planning out the kind of things you do in each week, can bring incredible powerful aligned focus to your BIG, BOLD, BEAUTIFUL soul goals and micro-actions.

Let's explore the Winter, Spring, Summer and Autumn seasons of each menstrual cycle:

Winter (days 1 – 6 of your cycle) – Menstruation, or the bleed phase. You might find yourself suited to things that don't take too much energy or concentration; you need to conserve your energy in this week. Taking the pause and space you need in your bleed week is a great start to working with your energy over the rest of the month. Do too much this week, and you could find yourself playing catch-up for the next three weeks!

Things to do in your Winter week:

- Rest!
- Plan the month ahead
- Set intentions
- Connect to your intuition and creativity

Spring (days 7 – 14) – Estrogen and testosterone (the get shit done hormones) start to rise and you start feeling the good vibes. Day 14 is usually where ovulation occurs if you have a 28-day cycle. This is your peak week, where you might find yourself wanting to create collaborative opportunities, work on something you've been stuck on, or get yourself out into the world.

Things to do in your Spring week:

- Work on complex tasks
- Get creative

- Get networking – reach out to new contacts and explore collaborative opportunities
- Launch something you've been working on

Summer (days 15 – 22) – The hazy, crazy days of summer. This week in your cycle is where, after your ovulation days, your estrogen and testosterone hormones take a natural dive and progesterone rises. The sedative qualities can make you feel a little quieter and more reflective. This is a great time for writing and creativity. You might find it a good time to analyse data or review information you've been gathering. Although, this week can leave you with brain fog toward the end of it.

Things to do in your Summer week:

- Group work
- Attend events / meetings
- Be proactive in pushing forward on a project
- Have difficult conversations (because this is the week when your confidence tends to be higher)

Autumn (days 23 – 28) – Otherwise known as your pre-menstrual week, this is when most of your hormones are leaving town until you go through your next bleed cycle. You might find you have a burst of energy to get shit done as your body prepares to close the doors for your bleed. A little like getting the house ready for nesting and hunkering down for the winter season! This can be a productive week for cleaning, decluttering or organizing. Be mindful that this week is likely to play with your mojo, and you can be more negative and cynical. Treat yourself kindly, and don't go throwing all your great work in the bin, because your inner critic is more than likely to be having the kind of party that you don't want to be invited to in this week! It's not all bad though – this can be the perfect week for looking back on the month that's been, and reviewing what's worked well, and what you want to put in place for your next month. It's also a great time to edit and review anything you've been working on because your critical eyes act as a pretty good BS detector for anything that your Spring/Summer self might have been writing cheques for that your ass can't cash!

Things to do in your Autumn week:

- Solo reflective work
- Decluttering, clearing and organizing your space
- Clearing out your email inbox and answering anything you've not yet got to
- Reviewing / editing work
- Study and learning

Of course, energy and cycles vary from person to person and from month to month, or year to year. There are many complex factors that cause fluctuations and changes in your hormone production and your energy levels, such as perimenopause, diabetes, thyroid issues, adrenal fatigue and polycystic ovary syndrome. Only you can get to know your body and your energy levels so you can work with them. The best way to do this is to track your cycle, notice how you are feeling on a week-by-week basis, and figure out what kind of tasks work best for you.

Some of the things you can start by tracking in each season are:

- Energy levels
- Mood / emotions
- How sociable / anti-social you feel
- What tasks worked well for you in that week
- What tasks didn't work well for you in that week

Using the Moon's lunar cycle as a pattern of productivity

If you don't have a menstrual cycle, or your periods are very irregular, you can still follow this pattern of cyclical productivity by working with the Moon's lunar cycle. This aligned lunar cycle is broken down as follows:

● New Moon = Winter (days 1 – 6)
◑ First Quarter = Spring (days 7 – 13)
○ Full Moon = Summer (days 14 – 21)
◐ Last Quarter = Autumn (days 22 – 28)

WORKING WITH YOUR OWN ENERGY

It goes without saying that everything shared here is unique to you. The idea is that when you get to know more about how you best work in alignment with yourself, you can bear the most fruit in terms of working on your BIG, BOLD, BEAUTIFUL soul goals.

The most important thing is to start getting really curious about your own energy in relation to your circadian rhythms, the waves of your ultradian rhythms and the might and wisdom of menstrual or moon cycles. You do you. That can never be wrong!

A FINAL WORD ON THOSE SHINY SQUIRRELS

The sure-fire way that you will create most leverage and momentum in working with your BIG, BOLD, BEAUTIFUL soul goals is to stay in true alignment with them by bringing them into being with focus, attention and action.

The thing to keep reminding yourself of is the 90- and 30-day goals you are working toward, and even the daily or weekly micro-actions you've set out for yourself. These will take you to those one-degree shift steps on your BIG, BOLD, BEAUTIFUL life adventure. And while things will come along, and opportunities will present themselves (like magic, sometimes!), if you find that you're getting excited by a million different ideas, remember they aren't always things you should do, or even need to do.

As Elizabeth Gilbert shares in her book *Big Magic: Creative Living Beyond Fear,* ideas are alive and they will seek an available collaborator in human form. Like lightning they will try and find a way to conduct themselves into being through us. Whether we choose to make all of those ideas happen in a week, or in a lifetime, is down to us.

This is why now when I have those seemingly ground-breaking, life-changing ideas in the shower, I make note of them and give them space to breathe before I take action. I will look at them in alignment with my BIG, BOLD, BEAUTIFUL soul goals. I'll think about what I have coming up, and decide whether it goes into the "take action now" pot of productivity, or a "not for now" space.

In fact, some of my ideas have become a BIG, BOLD, BEAUTIFUL reality *because* I have given them the space, focus and attention they deserved. And some of those other ground-breaking, life-changing ideas, which were jumping up and down to get my attention, show up for what they really are … simply an idea, rather than a shiny squirrel that would take my attention from the current wonderful thing I'm working on!

As you have explored in this step, finding focus goes deeper than just sitting down and drafting out that never ending to-do list; there's science and practical application to bringing focus to your BIG, BOLD, BEAUTIFUL soul goals.

STEP TWO REVIEW TIME

This has been the step where your BIG, BOLD, BEAUTIFUL vision and soul goals take off on the journey to start bringing it all into BIG, BOLD, BEAUTIFUL being. Action is where the magic starts becoming a reality, and it's important to revisit this step often to keep you continue crafting your actions and momentum as you move forward.

In this step you have:

✓ Uncovered where you've been *over-complicating things* and how you can shift from overwhelm to opportunity when working on your soul goals.

✓ Learned about the *power of the one-degree shift and aligned micro-actions* that will help you create and keep momentum each and every day.

✓ Figured out how to turn that momentum into action, *ditching the distractions by creating 90-day and 30-day focus plans,* to get you organized and on your way.

✓ Learned about your *biological rhythms and flows,* so that you can work *in alignment with your energy* to breathe life into your actions and soul goals, rather than burning out and giving up!

Now that you've explored how to bring your BIG, BOLD, BEAUTIFUL soul goals into action and focus, it's time to move onto STEP THREE … the one where you meet resistance face on, and work to bust beyond it rather than let it pour water on your BIG, BOLD, BEAUTIFUL dreams.

Of course before you dive straight on into STEP THREE, now is a natural time to take a break, so head on over for your BIG, BOLD, BEAUTIFUL breakout ritual to play with pendulum power, and learn how to get a deeper connection to your intuitive inner wisdom.

BREAKOUT RITUAL
SEVEN STEPS TO PENDULUM POWER

It's completely natural to find yourself getting in a head-spin at certain points as you move forward with your BIG, BOLD, BEAUTIFUL soul goals. If you do find yourself trapped by indecision, using a pendulum is a great way to finding the answers you've been searching for. They work with your own energy and intuition, and connect to your subconscious mind to tune into the answers you've been searching for, but have maybe got stuck on.

Pendulums are something made from either wood, metal or crystal and attached to a string or chain. When programmed they can answer a "yes" or "no" question.

HOW TO START WORKING WITH A PENDULUM

1. *Before you get started*
   - You can make a pendulum by getting some string and a weighted object (stone, coin, crystal), or by using a pre-made pointed crystal or metal pendulum. This could also be a piece of jewellery such as a chain or a pendant.
   - Find somewhere quiet and free from distraction.
   - Light a candle and maybe some incense.
   - You might want some soft, instrumental music playing.
   - Set your intention for what you would like to receive as a result of working with your pendulum. This could be clarity on a certain subject or a clear decision on something.
   - Be open and curious to whatever is ready to come through.

2. *Get in position*
   - Make sure you are seated as straight as possible with both feet on the floor.
   - Hold the chain or pendulum's fob between your thumb and forefinger.

- Arch your wrist slightly and steady your forearm. You will find it easier if your elbow is on something solid, like a table or the arm of a chair.
- Let the pendulum weight hang freely.
- If it's moving a lot, hold the weight until it's still, then gently let go. (Don't worry if your hand shakes a little; it won't affect the outcome.)

3. *Programme your answer signals*
   - Decide what your "yes", "no", "maybe" and "I don't know" signals are. Make sure they are clear.
   - This could be that the pendulum will swing up and down for "yes" (like a head nod) and side to side for "no" (like a head shake).
   - It could be that it swings in a straight line for "yes" and in a circular motion for "no".
   - It could be clockwise for "yes" and counter-clockwise for "no".
   - Tell your pendulum that these are the signals. Once you've done this a few times, you can skip this bit, as your pendulum will have been programmed to show you the answers this way.

4. *Check in on the signals*
   - To check that you are getting the right signal from your pendulum, ask a couple of questions to test out your signals.
   - You can ask anything from "Is my name X?", or "Is today Wednesday?"
   - These will verify the answer signals you've set.
   - If it's not working in the correct way, go back and reprogramme the pendulum, test and then continue.

5. *Ask your question*
   - Be as specific as you can when asking the question.
   - Make sure these are questions that have a "yes" or "no" answer. These could be related to specific action points from your soul goals that you want clarification on.

- For example, "Would I be better taking this action tomorrow?"; "Would it help me to speak to my boss about getting support on this project?"; "Is X the right person to be collaborating with?"; "Is this the best opportunity for me in relation to my overall vision?"

6. *Wait for the answer*
   - Be patient and keep bringing the question into your heart and mind. Don't rush to the answer.
   - Breathe deeply. You may find it helps to close your eyes.
   - Wait for the pendulum to start moving. If it doesn't, or the signal isn't clear, you can try rephrasing the question or simply asking again.
   - The pendulum may move a lot or it may be very slight. This could be related to the response – a clear, dynamic motion is a sign of big commitment, while a gentle movement might be a less whole-hearted response.

7. *Clear the pendulum*
   - At the end of asking the question you want an answer to, end the question by touching the pendulum weight to the palm of your hand or another surface, to signal that the question you asked has been answered.
   - You can move on to another question or draw this ritual to a close.

Using pendulums is a powerful energy check in when your head is getting stuck in overwhelm, or resistance, which you are going to explore in the next step!

STEP THREE

BUST BEYOND RESISTANCE

As you explored in STEP TWO, focus will help you take action toward your soul goals, so that you can start bringing that BIG, BOLD, BEAUTIFUL vision into crystal clear existence. That is, when you've ditched the distractions. Simple, right?

I'd love to tell you that you'll go sailing off into the sunset on your way to your BIG, BOLD, BEAUTIFUL vision board life, but the reality is that you are going to hit bumps in the road and roadblocks along the way, and the likelihood is that you're the one creating many of them!

GOOD INTENTIONS TURN TO DUST

What I have learned through years of holding space for those forging a path of living and creating a BIG, BOLD, BEAUTIFUL life (as well as from my own journey) is this ...

You will start off with a glitter cannon of excitement and motivation for what you are creating with your BIG, BOLD, BEAUTIFUL vision. You may notice the magic that starts coming your way, you will smash your actions and start celebrating the steps you are taking. And then ... the doubts will creep in, you will wonder if you've got what it takes, you will beat yourself up for having lost the loving feeling. You'll start to question whether the life you had before you started exploring your BIG, BOLD, BEAUTIFUL life was really that bad, and you might – just might – stop what you're doing and step back into that uncomfortable comfort zone, all while wishing things could be different.

This is resistance at play. It is real, and it is inevitable.

It will come along for the journey and can be an incredible opportunity for more self-awareness and growth. So, what better way to get equipped for it than getting to know it, and how you can work with it?

IN STEP THREE YOU WILL:

✓ Understand *your resistance habits* and how to gain awareness of any resistance patterns that will keep you wrapped up in an uncomfortable comfort zone, which could stop you making progress or taking action toward your soul goals.

✓ Get to know *what your fear and ego are really trying to tell you,* and how you can embrace the fact that every one of your behaviour patterns has a positive intention. Yes, that includes the ones that feel anything other than positive!

✓ Observe *resistance as a mind-body connection.* Recognize where and how resistance shows up in your body and brain, so you can help ease the tension when it arises, as you work on your soul goals.

✓ Understand *the difference between excitement and fear* and how to flip the script from disempowering to empowering language that will power up your actions and behaviours as you move forward.

✓ How to *get your brain on board and create the desire paths of connection* between thinking and doing, and how this can be a tool for life when it comes to creating momentum and acting on your soul goals.

✓ Why *behind every behaviour – even the ones that don't feel like they are serving you – there is a positive intention,* and when you know what that is, it's the key to unlocking wisdom to help you on your BIG, BOLD, BEAUTIFUL quest.

✓ How to start *moving beyond the fear of failure* and how you can have a positive relationship with failure to build creativity and resilience when working on your soul goals. I promise it's possible!

Oooheee, there's an incredible amount of BIG, BOLD, BEAUTIFUL wisdom for us to explore and move through in this powerful step, so let's get to it!

YOUR RESISTANCE HABITS

There is an absolute inevitability that resistance will tap you on the shoulder, or try and build a brick wall between you and your BIG, BOLD, BEAUTIFUL vision, as you use your soul goals to carve the path to making that vision a reality. Resistance is a physiological and psychological response to change. It happens every time you decide to do something different and step out of your comfort zone.

In order for you to create some impactful and positive changes, and manifest what you are bringing into BIG, BOLD, BEAUTIFUL being, things have to change. And change can feel daunting when you've spent so long doing things a certain way, thinking and behaving in ways that have been carved into your belief system, even if those thoughts, behaviours and beliefs have been the very things holding you back.

Think about it like a set of algorithms. Over the years your brain has learned the best and fastest way to avoid tricky situations. It's also figured out how to avoid danger and it thrives on being rewarded. When you are doing something that goes against these things, it's likely to kick up a whole lot of, "Hey! Hang on a hot minute ... That's not how we do things around here!" or, "What do you mean you want to live your best life? Can't we just have the one that we know?" to "Last time we did that, it didn't go well, did it?" or perhaps, "That looks like a whole lot of hard work. I'm not sure I can be bothered with that. Ooh ... a shiny squirrel!"

Your inner noise and chatter will be rumbling on in your mind. It will either support you, or sucker punch you. Some of it you may be aware of, some you won't have a clue about until you're getting going, only to find you're met with a stonewall of inaction and overwhelm.

You'll discover more about why this happens, and what's going on in your mind, body and brain in just a moment. But first, let's uncover how resistance shows up for you. Remember to look at this through the lens of curiosity and with the desire to create awareness of the things that could hold you back … because from awareness you can create different actions.

EXERCISE

IDENTIFY YOUR RESISTANCE HABITS

Take a look at these resistance habits. Put a tick by the ones that occur most often for you, and note *how* they show up.

☐ Procrastination

Example: "I will do anything other than the thing I have said I will work on. My oven/kitchen/bathroom/entire house has never been so clean."

....

....

☐ Over-complicating things

Example: "I often take a simple idea and add things to it until it becomes unrecognizable and feels completely impossible to achieve."

....

....

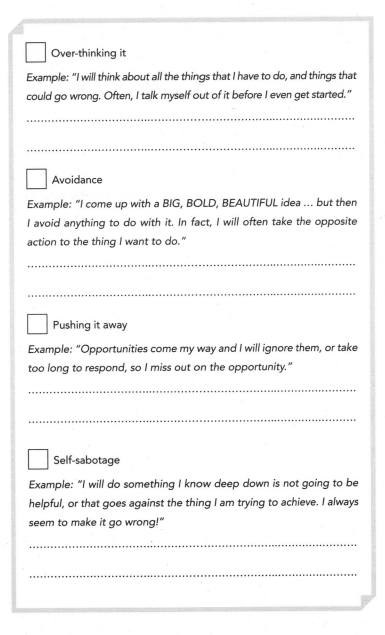

☐ Over-thinking it

Example: "I will think about all the things that I have to do, and things that could go wrong. Often, I talk myself out of it before I even get started."

....

....

☐ Avoidance

Example: "I come up with a BIG, BOLD, BEAUTIFUL idea ... but then I avoid anything to do with it. In fact, I will often take the opposite action to the thing I want to do."

....

....

☐ Pushing it away

Example: "Opportunities come my way and I will ignore them, or take too long to respond, so I miss out on the opportunity."

....

....

☐ Self-sabotage

Example: "I will do something I know deep down is not going to be helpful, or that goes against the thing I am trying to achieve. I always seem to make it go wrong!"

....

....

☐ Delay starting

Example: "I will leave things until the very last minute. Then, this huge amount of stress makes the whole process less enjoyable."

....

....

☐ Hitting the "f*ck it!" button

*Example: "I will go so far and take positive action, and then say 'F*ck it!', and undo all of my good work."*

....

....

☐ Perfectionism

Example: "I will put off doing something, or not take action, if it's not going to be perfect. If it's not perfect, I won't do it."

....

....

☐ Making excuses

Example: "I will come up with a million different reasons why it won't work out for me, or why I can't/shouldn't do it."

....

....

☐ Feeling stuck / inertia / low motivation and energy levels

Example: "I find it hard to get motivated, and feel too tired to start taking action."

....

....

☐ Fear of failure

Example: "I'm worried I'm going to get this so wrong that I will let people down, or they will think badly of me."

....

....

What themes have emerged? How are your resistance habits likely to show up when you're working toward something new?

Fill in the blanks ... "My main resistance habits show up as":

Example: "My main resistance habits show up as hitting the f*ck it button and continuing with negative behaviours that I know go against what I am trying to create in my BIG, BOLD, BEAUTIFUL life."

....

....

Now that you know this, what new habits can you create? Take this over to your journal or notepad to come up with some new resistance habits. *Example: "I can feel when the f*ck it button is ready to get hit. Instead of automatically going with it, I am going to take a deep breath, count to 10 and connect with the BIG, BOLD, BEAUTIFUL vision of what I am creating."*

As you've now gained awareness on your resistance habits, you can take this forward and bring this awareness with you to understand what's at play when you get caught in the resistance leg trap, and just what you can do to bring yourself out of it.

THE ROLE OF FEAR & EGO IN REACHING YOUR SOUL GOALS

I would love to tell you that, once you are clear on where you're going in your BIG, BOLD, BEAUTIFUL life, everything ahead of you is all angels riding unicorns over rainbows. It's not. There are going to be things that fall in your path on this journey and to try to throw you off track. It's good to know what they are before we get going.

Step in fear and ego ...

It's important that we talk about fear and ego and how they are the root cause of resistance. They will try and stop you, or trip you up, at different times and in different ways. They will kick up: before you've started, when you set your vision, while you are on your way, halfway through, and even when you're on the path toward your BIG, BOLD, BEAUTIFUL life. In fact, they will be along for every step of the ride.

So, let's get that conscious awareness ...

When I talk about ego throughout the book, I might interchange it with your "inner critic" or "inner dialogue". Let's uncover what they are, and how you can work with them.

Fear pops up whenever you are creating and making new plans. It wants to keep you safe. Ego wants certainty and proof, even though nothing is truly certain, and the only proof you will have is when you do the thing you are creating in your BIG, BOLD, BEAUTIFUL life. Does that mean you shouldn't do it? Oh, hell no! But your ego and fear will pop up and tell you stories about why you shouldn't in case everything goes horribly wrong. Ever wanted to do something new, and you immediately get the "what ifs" bubble up?

WHAT IS EGO?

Rather than how confident or arrogant someone is, ego is an inner sense of self-regulation. It's how you think about yourself, how you relate to the world around you, and your role and identity in the world. Your ego is essentially like wearing a big pair of sunglasses through which you see the world, the part you play, and what you project onto your view of the world.

The ego is your check-in point – a mediator between your desires and the real world. It relies on reason and stability to make sure you don't throw your life into chaos at any given moment. It also scrutinizes your moral conduct and behaviour, making sure that you don't act so outrageously that you get thrown out of the herd and are left to fend for yourself, which is what human survival has been based upon.

Basically, your ego likes to keep you on the straight and narrow. It wants to keep you safe, so will seek out certainty and control, to make sure you don't go on completely wild and dangerous tangents. Your ego loves donning the metaphorical pyjamas and slippers for a cosy night in. It will keep you in a comfort zone even when it's no longer comfortable to be there!

It's not all strict schoolmaster, though. When you are working with ego in a healthy way (see p. 84) it can keep you focused, flexible and motivated. It's also great at making sure you're staying in alignment with your values.

THE ROLE OF FEAR

Fear is a response to the ego, which results in the creation of wild scenarios within, which fill your imagination with what could possibly go wrong. It's no wonder it can take the shine off your BIG, BOLD, BEAUTIFUL vision. Left unchecked it can become the driving force that derails your BIG, BOLD, BEAUTIFUL plans.

Fear is natural. It plays an evolutionary role, making sure that we survive as a species. On an individual level fear plays a fundamental role in making sure you don't wipe out the course of your life. Of course, we don't have the clear and present danger of man-eating animals on every street corner these days, but we do have the fear that we are going to fail or fuck things up. And the physical, mental and emotional response is still as real today as it was 200,000 years ago.

Both ego and fear have one objective, which is to keep you safe. It's just that when you are making moves forward with your BIG, BOLD, BEAUTIFUL life, and they sense changes that make everything seem chaotic and uncertain, they throw up a heady (and physical) combination of wobbles that can make you wonder why you set about wanting to change things in the first place.

Your fear and ego responses might show up as:

Resistance	Self-sabotage
Confusion	Hiding
Apathy	Freezing
Procrastination	Negative self-talk
Anxiety	Doubt in yourself
Imposter syndrome	Doubt in what you're doing
Negative comparison	Doubt in this work
to others	Doubt in me!

WAYS TO WORK *WITH* YOUR EGO AND FEAR

The most important thing is to be aware of fear and ego and make sure they don't go unchecked. Otherwise, they will take you off into a spin cycle of overwhelm and doubt, picking up all the reasons you shouldn't do the thing you really want to do.

Bringing awareness, self-compassion and self-care together as you go through every move toward your BIG, BOLD, BEAUTIFUL life will help you to become stronger and resilient with each step out of your comfort zone.

Here are some powerful ways to help when fear and ego are trying to take control of the steering wheel.

1. Acknowledge it

Awareness and acknowledgement are the first steps to a positive solution. Don't try and ignore your fear, repress it or push it down, because the likelihood is that it will crop up in another way ... or shout 10 times louder if you're not taking any notice of it. Instead, acknowledge it's there, and try to identify the trigger points that cause it to arise.

2. Create a doorSTOP

There are around 100 milliseconds, just one-tenth of a second, before a thought of something daunting signals to the brain to create a fear response. Once that fear button has been pushed it creates a dialogue in the mind that is all fear based. 100 milliseconds may not sound like a long time, but it is enough to put a doorstop between the fear trigger and the cascade of unhelpful thought vomit. I like to use a mindful practice called the STOP technique as a way to stop fear having the ultimate buzzkill party.

It's simple and easy to implement, and it goes like this:

STOP. When the thoughts start bubbling up, stop what you are doing. Don't go with them ... STOP. This will create a natural pause between the fear and the thoughts.

Take a breath. Breathe three deep inhales and exhales to bring your brain and body back into balance.

Observe. Reflect on why these thoughts might be coming up. Don't judge them; be curious. What does your fear want you to know that could be useful information? Come up with three simple things you need to be reminded of, or solutions, that will help you.

Example: "My fear is letting me know that I could go into burnout if I do too much. So I will keep my goals simple. I will remind myself that I don't have to rush and that I can take my time.

Proceed by taking any useful information, or actions, and moving forward.

The truth is that a lot of your thought patterns are based on things that happened to you between your formative ages of two to seven years old. This is the age at which our beliefs are set. If you had a negative experience related to your sense of self, or to your abilities to do things, then this will be with you whenever you are trying to do something. You are likely having the same emotional response now as you did at the age you were when it first happened.

You wouldn't get angry or frustrated at a child for having a fear response and you certainly wouldn't call it stupid. You would try to make that child feel safe and assured. It's the same with your fear.

Get curious; ask it what it's afraid of. Becoming an observer of the fear means it can no longer run the show and throw a fear party. Journal on what comes up, with a big serving of compassion and understanding.

Ask your fear what it needs right now to feel safe. It might tell you to take things a little slower, or that it needs to know what you'll do if things don't go according to plan. I like to think of this as creating a safety blanket to wrap around fear. Then, you can respond in a helpful way. It could be giving you some pragmatic and practical pull chords to use if things don't go the way you expected.

Burnout, stress, overwhelm and certain phases of your Moon or menstrual cycle can make things feel more unmanageable than they actually are. Fear will respond. Become aware of what you need to do for self-care 101 in that moment to help you as you are taking action on your BIG, BOLD, BEAUTIFUL soul goals.

RESISTANCE AND THE MIND BODY CONNECTION

Resistance isn't just something that knocks on your door and shows up as the buzzkill to your vibes when you are disco dancing away on the path your BIG, BOLD, BEAUTIFUL vision map is taking you.

Resistance comes up because there are signals saying that change is a-coming and it doesn't feel safe. As humans we're hard-wired to opt for safety over danger and stability over the drama of the unknown. Our bodies and brains are literally built to make sure that, as a species, we stay on this planet for as long as possible (even when some of our collective behaviours imply otherwise!). So when change comes along, your mind and body's spidey senses will go on high alert, and kick in the chat that sends signals through the body to say … "Hmmm, are we sure about this? I'm not too keen on these new-fangled BIG, BOLD, BEAUTIFUL changes you're making." Then, BOOM! In comes resistance to shut it down, stat!

Like understanding *how* your resistance behaviours and habits show up, recognizing how resistance shows up in your body can help you gain awareness of when it's happening and what you can do to ease your reaction when it does.

These are some of the ways resistance can show up physically in the body:

- Muscle tension in the neck, shoulders, jaw, joints. Tightness in the shoulders can mean you are carrying too much emotional load. Resistance in your knees can mean the inability to move forward.
- Headache, eye strain and tension in the head. This can mean over-thinking, tension, the stress of not getting things underway, or worrying about what will happen if you do or don't take action.
- Knots in the stomach, butterflies, sweating, heart palpitations, upset stomach, cold sweats, shortness of breath, IBS and digestive issues. These are physical manifestations of anxious feelings.

- Brain fog is not being able to think straight, or lacking the concentration or focus to be able to work on the actions you've set out for yourself.
- Feeling fatigued, drained and exhausted, and with little motivation, like you haven't got the physical or emotional bandwidth to be able to do anything.
- Being overstimulated with too much energy, feeling jittery, wired, unable to hold a thought together.

How does resistance show up for you physically? In other words, what are your physical resistance symptoms?
Example: "I feel heavy in my shoulders and have tension in my neck and shoulders."

....

....

How do you become aware resistance is happening?
Example: "I get a pain in my neck that feels like I've slept awkwardly, but doesn't go away, even after a couple of days."

....

....

What could you do to help ease the tension around resistance?
Example: "Self-massage for muscle tension, affirmations or breathing exercises to help with anxious feelings, moving my body if I don't have enough physical energy (shaking or dancing is great for this)."

....

....

FEAR VS. EXCITEMENT: FLIPPING THE SCRIPT

The truth of the matter is that when you are creating change, even if it is for things that you most want in your BIG, BOLD, BEAUTIFUL life your body will send up the danger flare by activating the sympathetic nervous system – your fight or flight response – and that comes with physiological and psychological stimuli.

To add to the complexity of everything that's going on under the surface, fear and excitement basically have the same physiological responses of butterflies, tummy flips, heart racing, shortness of breath, nausea, upset stomach, feeling jittery … it goes on.

So, if you know that fear and excitement are basically two sides of the same coin, how can you work with the feelings to bust beyond resistance, rather than letting the fear flip itself up higher on the seesaw of emotions?

One way to work with fear and excitement is to think about them like the "move away from" and "move toward" energy you explored in STEP ONE (pp. 16–18).

Fear is "move away from", meaning you don't want the experience you are creating from your BIG, BOLD, BEAUTIFUL vision and soul goals.

Excitement, on the other hand, is "move toward" – meaning you are welcoming in this aspect of what you are creating from your BIG, BOLD, BEAUTIFUL vision and soul goals.

EXERCISE

GET TO KNOW THE DIFFERENCE BETWEEN FEAR AND EXCITEMENT

When you are working on your BIG, BOLD, BEAUTIFUL actions, and you experience a physiological response, take a pause and check in with yourself.

Ask yourself these two simple questions, check in with any physiological or psychological responses, and write out what comes up.

1. Is what I'm working on right now something that I want to move away from?
   Yes/No
   Example: "It feels fraught with danger, and ultimately unsafe."

2. Is what I'm working on right now something I am moving toward?
   Yes/No
   Example: "It feels exciting and a little scary, but ultimately it's what I want."

If you answered "yes" to the first question then fear and anxiety may become overwhelming. It may be time to re-evaluate whether what you're working on really is right for you, or what you need to do to make it feel less terrifying if it holds no real danger for you.

If you answer "yes" to the second question, then you're likely to be experiencing the feels of excitement. You can work with these by powering how you speak to yourself about the actions you're taking, flipping the script on the fear voice.

You can do this by:

- Acknowledging the feelings
- Flipping the script
- Reframing into something positive

Here are a couple of examples:

"Even though I'm feeling a huge amount of feelings about going for this promotion, I'm excited to talk to my boss about the opportunities it could create, both for me and for my career."

"Even though I feel butterflies in my tummy when I think about that presentation, and standing up in front of people to give it, I am excited about conveying my message and creating some new connections that can help me raise my profile."

Try it out for yourself:

Even though I'm feeling ....

....

I'm excited by ....

....

Even though I'm feeling ....

....

I'm excited by ....

....

Now you've completed this exercise, you should have a good idea of when to honour the excitement, even though there is discomfort (because what's on the other side is ultimately rewarding), and when to be aware that fear is in the house and how you might flip the script on it.

As you explore more self-empowerment and self-care in STEPS FIVE and SIX, you will learn more tools to build confidence, and compassion to help you build in more resilience and wellbeing into your BIG, BOLD, BEAUTIFUL journey.

GET YOUR BRAIN ON BOARD
WITH YOUR SOUL GOALS

It's not just thoughts, behaviours, beliefs and physiology that have to move with changes in order to make them happen. Your whole mind and body need to get with the programme too, especially your brain.

During your childhood and teenage years, your brain goes on a wild ride creating all the neural pathways, or communication paths, that send signals between different parts of the nervous system. They transmit information for learning, growing and developing. By the age of 25 your adult brain has pretty much fully developed … and so has the way you think, act, behave and feel.

Throughout this huge period of growth these communication paths create your belief systems. These form habits, biases, attitudes and so much more. It can be harder to change habits and behaviours past 25, but it's not impossible.

YOUR BRAIN AND NEUROPLASTICITY

The neural communication connections in the brain are plastic (neuroplasticity), meaning that they are flexible and can change as a result of behaviours, to create new empowering habits. So much of what you will be learning and experiencing in each of the seven steps in this book will help you to build neuroplasticity. It is the brain's natural ability to change by creating new neural pathways and clearing away those which are no longer used.

I like to think of it like this …

Think about a field that's has been walked over so many times, there's a natural path that's been worn down from one side of the field to the other – this is called a desire path. Your neurotransmitters do the same thing – they carry information to different points in your brain by travelling across well-trodden desire paths. This is how habits are formed, and the basal ganglia part of the brain, which is responsible for motor learning, executive functions, behaviours and emotions, loves habit.

Building neuroplasticity will help you move beyond the confines of those uncomfortable comfort zones. It will keep your brain curious, intuitive and open to creating new pathways that are in alignment with your BIG, BOLD, BEAUTIFUL soul goals. This requires you to create new habits and form new neural desire paths that encourage positive and empowering habits. You will need to stretch yourself and take empowered action.

It's time to go to the brain gym!

Living BIG, BOLD and BEAUTIFULLY builds brain plasticity.

Research undertaken by Joyce Shaffer at the University of Washington has shown that the key things needed to keep the brain plastic are: challenge, novelty and focused attention.

This is great news for all things BIG, BOLD and BEAUTIFUL because:

1. CHALLENGE

Creating those moves toward BIG, BOLD, BEAUTIFUL goals with soul will stretch you beyond your comfort zones. You will forge into the wild unknown, doing things that excite and inspire you.

2. NOVELTY

When you are trying out new things, going on adventures of mind, body and soul and doing things you've never done before, this is all new and novel. You might be meeting new people, going to new places, experiencing a variety of cultures, or learning different skills. As a result your brain will problem-solve and adapt; those neurons will fire up new ways to adapt to new experiences.

3. FOCUSED ATTENTION

As you explored in STEP TWO, finding focus will help you move toward your BIG, BOLD, BEAUTIFUL vision. As you are focusing on each step, and every one-degree shift, you are building stronger desire paths and forming habits that make your possibilities an inevitability.

FOR EVERY BEHAVIOUR THERE IS A POSITIVE INTENTION

OK, so this is a little bit of a mind bender, so bear with me on this one. I promise you if you can get behind it then it really can blow resistance out of the water.

Understanding and becoming aware of your behaviours and what's behind them is great, but what if I were to tell you that every behaviour has a positive intention, even when it might appear that it's anything but? From procrastination, or over-complicating your soul goals, through to behaviours such as smoking. Yes, really! I'll explain more in a moment.

And what if, when you understand what that intention is, you can then use that knowledge to help support your BIG, BOLD, BEAUTIFUL growth?

Sounds good, but still not sure?

I like to think of this as the "wholeness of life". We often say it about ourselves – "On one hand I'm this, and on the other hand I'm this." We are constantly playing with duality. You might be thinking and feeling something along the lines of, "On one hand I feel excited about my BIG, BOLD, BEAUTIFUL vision and goals, but on the other hand I'm worried I might not have what it takes to make it happen/I'm afraid of what will happen when I do/it all seems like a lot of hard work, and I'm knackered!"

You might find yourself wanting to take action with all of your heart, and then finding yourself taking none at all. The behaviour might look like avoidance or fear, but the *positive intention of* this behaviour is to not overwhelm your system.

You might want to create healthy habits. Let's take giving up smoking as an example – you really want to give up, but you're finding it almost impossible to give up the habit of smoking. Of course, there's more to it when it comes to giving up an addiction to nicotine in this case, but what's underneath the unhealthy habit could be the *positive intention of* taking time to pause out of your hectic day; perhaps, smoking gives you the chance to do that.

Personally, my particular go-to behaviour is to pile more and more work onto my plate, creating new and exciting projects that take up all my time, energy and attention. The *positive intention* is that I am constantly evolving and creating new things, which means I am meeting my soul's purpose.

The behaviour leads to a pay-off of some kind, so you need to make sure that it's still met in some way. Becoming aware of the *positive intention* underlying seemingly negative behaviours, is like having the secret code to unlock information that can help you to unpick the resistance behaviour. Once you've done this you can work with it to support your BIG, BOLD, BEAUTIFUL journey.

Try this out to get down with your positive intentions and work with them.

EXERCISE

DISCOVER THE POSITIVE INTENTIONS BEHIND THE BEHAVIOURS

BIG, BOLD, BEAUTIFUL SOUL GOAL	RESISTANCE BEHAVIOUR	POSITIVE INTENTION UNDERPINNING THE RESISTANCE BEHAVIOUR	THE LEARNING THAT WILL SUPPORT & MOVE ME TOWARD MY BIG, BOLD, BEAUTIFUL SOUL GOAL
Example: To feel healthy and strong to support what I am creating in my BIG, BOLD, BEAUTIFUL life. This means sticking to a regular form of exercise and eating well.	Eating foods that don't necessarily support a healthy lifestyle.	To feel fulfilled and enjoy something I get pleasure from.	I can find exercise that I find fulfilling and enjoy, and I can still enjoy some of those treats mindfully. Call the smaller weights at the gym donuts to associate them with the enjoyment of food!* (*This one really works for me!)

BIG, BOLD, BEAUTIFUL SOUL GOAL	RESISTANCE BEHAVIOUR	POSITIVE INTENTION UNDERPINNING THE RESISTANCE BEHAVIOUR	THE LEARNING THAT WILL SUPPORT & MOVE ME TOWARD MY BIG, BOLD, BEAUTIFUL SOUL GOAL

MOVING BEYOND THE FEAR
OF FAILURE

This one is a biggie for combatting resistance. I would say the number one challenge that most people who are walking the BIG, BOLD, BEAUTIFUL path have to contend with is our old nemesis ... failure.

It's the thing my clients have to hold the stare with time and time again on the BIG, BOLD, BEAUTIFUL journey.

Failure is where the "what ifs" live:

What if I do this and it all goes horribly wrong like the last time?
Cue memories of what happened the last time you did something that didn't work out and you felt ashamed/embarrassed/insert big feeling here.

What if I leave my paid job to venture out on this new business idea and I lose a regular salary?
Cue disaster movie scenarios of ending up homeless and penniless, or having to tell your family that you f*cked up big time.

What if I get so far with my BIG, BOLD, BEAUTIFUL soul goals, people don't get it and judge me, or leave me?
Cue doing something that leads to feelings of isolation, judgement, being shunned, not feeling like you belong.

These feelings are all valid, and will be rumbling on under the surface, to the point where the idea of failing becomes bigger than the desire to create your BIG, BOLD, BEAUTIFUL vision, and will bring things to a thunderous halt.

But before you close this book at the seemingly overwhelming enormity of failure, I want you to know that you absolutely can move beyond the fear of failing. You can even have a positive relationship with it – one that builds creativity, allows you to take measured risks and builds resilience, which are some of the key ingredients of busting beyond resistance and creating movement in your BIG, BOLD, BEAUTIFUL life.

The key to all of this is resilience. Resilience is something you are going to build as you step out of your comfort zones on this journey. And I can tell you, it is SO worth it, because what you learn about yourself – what you are capable of doing and being – will help you every time you set off on a new venture on your BIG, BOLD, BEAUTIFUL life. Because living a BIG, BOLD, BEAUTIFUL life is for life, not just for the pages of this book!

To put the BIG, the BOLD and the BEAUTIFUL into your plans you have to get creative – in every sense of the word. Creativity is the essence of crafting your BIG, BOLD, BEAUTIFUL soul goals and creating innovative ways to make them happen.

TAKING BIG, BOLD, BEAUTIFUL (MEASURED) RISKS

Measured risks are incredibly important, because it always takes risk to do something BIG, BOLD and BEAUTIFUL in your life … and as you do so, much of what you're doing is unknown, and with it brings an element of risk, which builds resilience.

The challenge is that most of us have been brought up to avoid risk at all costs. We've been taught that staying in our comfort zones, in our lane, is the safest place to be. The truth is that safety will keep you stagnant, whereas measured risk can bring both reward momentum, and a dash of excitement to keep things interesting.

So how do creativity, measured risk and resilience help you bust beyond the idea of failure? Creativity is never perfect; it's about trying things out (taking measured risks) and evolving ideas that haven't worked out (failure). Being resilient means not giving up at the first hurdle and developing on ideas.

Reframing thoughts and behaviours, to allow you to bust beyond resistance and bring failure into your journey, can actually become your best ally. To do this is to get down with the concept of Failing Forward – the idea that you allow a series of "failures" to happen in order to grow-learn-adapt. This in turn helps you to create momentum for your BIG, BOLD, BEAUTIFUL soul goals.

FAILING FORWARD

Failing forward is a concept widely known in leadership. It's where the conditions are created to allow mistakes and failures to be made, in order that what comes from the learning, helps to grow and develop the next stage or iteration of a project, product or idea.

Ed Catmull, one of the co-founders of creativity giant Pixar Inc., talks about the concept of failing forward as one of the key reasons they create such incredible outputs in their work. In his book *Creativity Inc.*, Catmull talks about failure being an inevitable and welcome (and if not welcome, then needed), part of the creative process.

> "Failure isn't a necessary evil. In fact, it isn't evil at all.
> It is a necessary consequence of doing something new."
> Ed Catmull

Moving beyond the fear of failure

Here are five of the key learnings from Catmull and failing forward that you get to bring into your BIG, BOLD, BEAUTIFUL process. Hopefully, they'll help you to keep busting through resistance:

1. *Create strong storytelling* – This is the embodied story of your BIG, BOLD, BEAUTIFUL vision. You have drawn a map of your future and what you are creating for your life.

2. *Be wrong as fast as you can* – Don't put things off because they are not perfect. Get things wrong, make mistakes quickly. Write the first shitty draft, take a first imperfect action, but take the action quickly and learn from it. Just do it!

3. *Create the containers for failing* – You get to create the space for failure and mistakes to happen. You get to create a beta version of something new and test it out. I do this every time I create a new course or programme. I start with a lite version of that course or programme, then invite a small test group to go through it, try it out and provide feedback on things that work well, and those that don't. From that space I can build out something based on the "failures" of the first iteration to create something that works better next time around.

4. *Have a disaster recovery plan* – Your ego isn't going to like it when you "fail". So, think of the things you can do to support your emotional wellbeing when you do, such as … having a community to support you for the wobbles and the wins, getting an accountability buddy, having a coach, having a solid self-care routine.

5. *You are not the failure* – Just because you have failed, this does not mean you are fundamentally flawed. It doesn't mean a single bloody thing about you, your ability, your value or your worth. Invite in the knowledge that failure is a piece of the jigsaw puzzle; it's a normal part of the process for things not to go to plan. This knowledge should allow you to turn pain into progress, taking comfort in the knowledge that there is a benefit from the growth that failure brings.

Taking these elements of failing forward, it's time to work out how you will put this into play when taking action on your BIG, BOLD, BEAUTIFUL soul goals.

EXERCISE

CREATE A PLAN FOR FAILING FORWARD

The BIG, BOLD, BEAUTIFUL story I am creating is …

Example: "I am creating a business from my creativity, which will give me the opportunity to explore and work on my own terms, and in my own way."

....

....

....

The first imperfect action I will take is …

Example: "I will send out a questionnaire to people I know who might be interested in what I want to offer. This will provide me with a raw, untested way to check in on the validity of my fledgling, un-researched idea in its initial state."

....

....

....

The failure containers I am going to create are …

Example: "I will send the questionnaire out to three people first to make sure I am asking the right questions, which will give me the information I need. Based on what comes back, I will change the questions if needed, or add more."

....

....

....

My disaster recovery plan is ...

Example: "I will give myself permission to change the idea if those three people think it is complete rubbish, and that I am crazy for even thinking it. I will also create affirmations that I am creative, flexible and full of inspirational ideas that help me and the people I am here to help."

....

....

....

I will remind myself that failure is part of the process by ...

Example: "Writing these affirmations out and having them where I can see them. I will breathe into how this feels in connection with my BIG, BOLD, BEAUTIFUL vision, so I can lift myself up and above anything that doesn't seem to go right, and stay connected to where I am heading."

....

....

....

The more you embrace the concept that "failing forward" (and all the other concepts you've explored in this step) are powerful tools that allow you to take the actions and steps on your BIG, BOLD, BEAUTIFUL journey, the less the grip the fear of failure has over you taking action, and resistance will melt away!

STEP THREE REVIEW TIME

So, here we are at the end of Step THREE: Bust Beyond Resistance. During this step you have moved through, and beyond, the energy that could keep you stuck in inaction. And you have learned *how* to move through it to power up the energy and action in your soul goals.

Here's a checklist that will give you an easy reference to come back when you feel resistance putting the blockers in place.

✓ Create awareness around your *resistance habits* and how they show up. Create new empowering habits that will support you instead of holding you back.

✓ Try the three mindful activities to work with fear and ego to create a more empowering narrative that will support you as you take action on your soul goals and progress on your BIG, BOLD, BEAUTIFUL journey.

✓ Recognize when *resistance shows up in your mind and body*, and explore further ways to help ease it.

✓ *Flip the script on fear,* turning it to excitement by shifting from disempowering to empowering inner dialogue.

✓ *Shift your resistance behaviour into positive action and intention,* which will support you as you work toward your BIG, BOLD, BEAUTIFUL soul goals.

✓ Create your *fail forward plan* to help support your BIG, BOLD, BEAUTIFUL soul goals. Or, try this any time resistance is showing up because of the fear that it's going to go wrong!

Now that you've busted beyond the resistance for the things that could hold you back from creating and living your BIG, BOLD, BEAUTIFUL life, it's time to move on to STEP FOUR, which is all about dialling up your energy to embody the expansion you are creating.

Before you do, now is a natural time to take a pause and reflect on what you've discovered in STEP THREE, so head on over to your BIG, BOLD, BEAUTIFUL breakout ritual, to create a beautiful elements release ritual to ground and connect.

BREAKOUT RITUAL
CREATING AN ELEMENTAL EARTH RELEASE RITUAL

So much of your resistance is related to the things you want to clear out of the way, or let go of, so that you can get to the action, energy and intention of your BIG, BOLD, BEAUTIFUL vision and soul goals.

This might be stories and narratives you're ready to move on from. It could be habits and behaviours that hold you back. Or it could be people and situations that you no longer physically have in your life, but they are energetically still connected to you, and you're ready to move on from them.

Creating a release ritual is a great way of energetically cutting the ties to the things that are not serving you. In this ritual you're going to connect to the earth, for slow and grounding release.

NATURE MANDALA

A mandala (meaning "circle" in Sanskrit) is a sacred geometrical shape that looks like a circle of patterns. It has been used as a form of meditation and devotion across many religions, such as Buddhism, Islam and Celtic paganism, for centuries. Creating a mandala as a form of earth offering for what you are releasing, transforms the "gifts" from all that you've learned from and are ready to let go of, and transforms the energy into something that nature uses as fuel and fertilizer.

You can create a mandala anywhere outdoors where you will leave it to do its work once your ritual is complete.

What you will need:

- Seeds
- Flowers & petals
- Stones
- Leaves, twigs or sticks
- Any other natural objects you can find, that you would like to add to your mandala

A quick note: It's important to use materials from the earth that you are offering the mandala to, so this could be materials you gather on a walk.

Create your nature mandala

- Start with a seed point in the middle of your mandala. As you plant the 'seed' in the centre of the mandala state what it is that you are releasing. This could be something significant that you are ready to say goodbye to.
- Create layers of your mandala by adding outward patterns from that central seed point using the flowers, leafs, or other objects you have collected.
- As you create the outward layers focus on what else you are releasing, or ready to say goodbye to.
- Create as many layers out from the central point as you wish, stating clearly what you are releasing, and saying goodbye with every layer.
- Once complete, spend a few moments in contemplation, along with the natural materials that have contributed to this offering, and gratitude for everything that is being released.
- Leave your mandala to break down naturally.

STEP FOUR

DIAL UP YOUR BIG, BOLD, BEAUTIFUL ENERGY

Now you've explored the ways in which you can work with – and through – resistance, it's time to meet the opposite to resistance: elevating your energy. In this step we will look at how you can harness some of the BIG, BOLD, BEAUTIFUL energy that is going to support and sustain you on your life-changing visionary quest.

The sure-fire way to bring long-lasting powerful change is to elevate and embody the energy of expansion you are creating with your BIG, BOLD, BEAUTIFUL vision and life.

When you take an aligned, empowered action you embody the energetic elevation of soul goals. You become the living, breathing manifestation or actualization of your BIG, BOLD, BEAUTIFUL vision.

Say your BIG, BOLD, BEAUTIFUL soul goals are to live and create from a life of freedom and adventure. You desire to do this through travel, finding a way to work from anywhere in the world that leads you to having adventures around the globe. Your life becomes the living embodiment of freedom and adventure.

ELEVATED ENERGY

Your BIG, BOLD, BEAUTIFUL life is that energetic connection to what you can create.

And energy is the connector in your embodiment journey. As you explored in STEP THREE, resistance is a mind-body connection that can hold you back from achieving your goals. Well, energy is also a mind-body connection which activates your BIG, BOLD, BEAUTIFUL vision and soul goals.

Elevated energy is the physical embodiment (somatic) of connection to your BIG, BOLD, BEAUTIFUL life. It is the catalyst to joy that powers you on all levels, and brings you into wellbeing balance. It does this through activating the parasympathetic nervous system, otherwise known as the "rest and digest" nervous system, a network of nerves that relaxes the body and brings it back into homeostasis (balance) after periods of stress, fear or danger. Not only is the parasympathetic nervous system vital for helping the body operate life-sustaining processes like digestion and repair – it also maintains mental and physical health by bringing the body to calm following stress reactions that cause increased blood pressure and heart rate, and divert energy from other body processes. Working with your parasympathetic nervous system when creating and working on your BIG, BOLD BEAUTIFUL vision and goals, will help your body and mind to feel resourceful, well and safe.

More than that, when you are truly connected and in alignment with mind, body and soul, then it's possible to tap into even more connected wisdom. Through this connection you can explore a deeper, more expansive, intuitively guided intelligence that becomes even more fuel for your BIG, BOLD, BEAUTIFUL journey.

This expansive, embodied, intuitively guided energy is going to be your life force to take your BIG, BOLD, BEAUTIFUL vision and soul goals to the next level. It's going to be your energetic wing buddy, to help you create bigger, be bolder and step into your beautiful adventures.

IN STEP FOUR YOU WILL:

✓ Discover the *wisdom of the body,* and why being in tune with your body will activate your energy to support your BIG, BOLD, BEAUTIFUL journey.

✓ Activate the *three brains in your body,* AKA *your body's intelligence centres,* to take your BIG, BOLD, BEAUTIFUL vision beyond an abstract concept. Learn how to work with each to create aligned energetic and embodied action toward your soul goals.

✓ Explore the *powerful vagus nerve, as the super-highway of connection* within your body that creates both the wellbeing runway and the energetic instruction manual for your BIG, BOLD, BEAUTIFUL vision.

✓ *Become a vibrational match* for your BIG, BOLD, BEAUTIFUL vision and soul goals, and ultimately your BIG, BOLD BEAUTIFUL life, by activating the power of #alreadydone to manifest energetic inevitability.

✓ Explore how your words, actions and behaviours matter and *how to model and embody your energetic elevation* to dial your energy up and be in the energetic alignment of the vision and goals you created way back in STEP ONE.

✓ And finally, activate the *simple power of JOY,* and how to bring more of it into daily being.

Get ready to create some next level expansive energy in your BIG, BOLD, BEAUTIFUL journey.

Don your sequin cape, and get ready to vibe fly!

YOUR BODY IS INFINITELY WISE

Let's face it; it can be all too easy to spend time thinking rather than being when it comes to this BIG, BOLD, BEAUTIFUL journey of a lifetime. The inevitable truth is that you can – and you will – overthink, over-plan, and over-complicate it.

I share this from my own tendencies and behaviours, and the hard-way-round way I used to do things before finding the BIG, BOLD, BEAUTIFUL path. I'm a massive over-thinker and over-planner. Some of this has to do with perfectionist tendencies, which I have to constantly work with … Oh yes, I see yours too. And there's a whole heap of stories and narratives I can make up in my head about why I'm not good enough, or capable enough. You get them too? Most of us do.

And then there's the people-pleasing. Oooeeee, is there the people pleasing! I'm not a recovered people pleaser yet, but I do recognize it, and I am working on it.

I spent a long time being stuck in my head – years and years in fact. When it came to doing, I was there with the best of them. I could strategize, plan, act, do, then rinse and repeat ad infinitum. You might think that sounds OK. I mean, it's still *doing,* after all … but all that doing is a high-speed train to overwhelm and burnout, which seems to be something of an epidemic of our time.

I know we've been talking a lot about taking action, but it's important to be aware that spending all your time doing actually hinders your BIG, BOLD, BEAUTIFUL progress. Instead of it feeling fun and exciting, it starts to feel like a slog, or you lose interest because you're spending more time thinking and doing all the things and what you want still seems so out of reach.

This generally happens when you've disconnected from the full embodied experience of what a BIG, BOLD, BEAUTIFUL life gets to truly be. Connecting to the powerful experiences this journey can bring means being present to it. That's impossible when all that's happening exists only in your never-ending to-do list.

It takes work – and a fair amount of unlearning the unhelpful habits and behaviours you may have adopted throughout life – but one of the key ways to shift from doing to being is by connecting to the full wisdom of the body. This means getting out of your head, and exploring the infinite wisdom of the body, to support your BIG, BOLD, BEAUTIFUL journey.

Dropping from the thinking mind into the feeling body can reveal emotional patterns, energy shifts and incredible opportunities for transformation that will not only support your BIG, BOLD, BEAUTIFUL journey, but will become an essential part of existing and being within your BIG, BOLD, BEAUTIFUL life.

WHAT IS BODY WISDOM?

As humans we have innate body wisdom. This wisdom, or "somatic intelligence", has evolved over millennia. It has kept us safe from danger, it has helped us forage for food and it has helped us form bonds with others so that we can mate, thrive in a community, and find a sense of belonging.

This wisdom is a constant dialogue, running between body and mind. On the most fundamental level your body will communicate with you when it's tired, hungry, too hot or too cold, when it doesn't feel safe, when it feels stressed, or when it feels relaxed. This dialogue is happening 24 hours a day, even when you're asleep as your body does its housekeeping to repair, recharge and replenish.

The challenge we have in our "always on" culture is that there are signal disruptors that get in the way of paying attention to our body's innate wisdom. You can disrupt and bypass your natural rhythms to work longer and harder. You no longer have to hunt for food because it's instantly available, which means you can bypass the body's natural hunger signals. Technology means you can work from anywhere in the world, at any time of night and day, and in any time zone, so you can push on through fatigue or exhaustion.

All this bypassing and living in an over-stimulated, noisy world, can make it so much more difficult to be in tune with your body and its innate wisdom. But it is possible through some of the embodiment and somatic practices we will explore in this step (and for your BIG, BOLD BEAUTIFUL journey).

I can with full, hand on heart (see, it's even in the language of the body!) say that connecting the wisdom of my body through somatic awareness and connection was the turning point of unlocking the treasure chest of wisdom in my body, and this work. I'm excited that we're going to explore this together.

THE BODY'S INTELLIGENCE CENTRES, AKA THE THREE BRAINS

Body intelligence is ancient wisdom. Somatic embodiment practices such as yoga, Qoya, tai chi, qigong, the Alexander Technique and Pilates, work with the body's innate wisdom to explore how the body feels, and the powerful knowledge it has within. When you experience what's within you body, rather than how your body might be viewed, you get into an incredible relationship within your life from the inside out.

We are now in a place where Western medicine, technology and neuroscience have advanced enough to prove that some of the ancient embodiment teachings of yoga, tai chi and qigong are based on scientific fact.

One of the more recent scientific discoveries of somatic wisdom is that the body has three "brains": head, heart and gut. Each have complex neural networks, which communicate with each other and store and process information in different ways. When you work with all three, you can create with them, and bring them together to bring a more aligned experience to your BIG, BOLD, BEAUTIFUL journey. Basically, getting all of yourself in the game! Each also has the ability for neuroplasticity, which – as we discovered in STEP THREE – is the ability to rewire and create new neural pathways – essential for growth and development to support you on all levels of your BIG, BOLD, BEAUTIFUL journey,

It's time to get all of your brains and body in on the BIG, BOLD, BEAUTIFUL action. Let's explore the three brains:

The head brain (the cephalic brain) is made up of 100 billion brain cells, otherwise known as neurons or information messengers. It is both analytical and logical, meaning that it works on data and reasoning to function. The head brain processes information based on this data, and will look at the "information" it is presented with objectively and with rationality. This is why you will often find that those beautiful moments of inspiration and creativity soon get over-taken with planning, strategy, logic and reason. This is your head brain running the show.

Here are some examples of the way the head brain communicates:
   "I think"
   "Logically speaking"
   "Rationally speaking"
   "Intellectually I know that"
   "The plan is …"

The heart brain (the cardiac brain) is made up of 40,000 neurons. As well as its key function, which is to keep you alive by pumping blood and oxygen around your body, it acts as a transmitter to feel, sense, learn and remember the world in you, and around you. It is where memories and big feelings are held. Just try this little experiment for a moment ... Think for a moment of a time when you have experienced a feeling of deep connection to something, maybe love, sadness or joy; where would you put your hand on your body as you connect into this memory or feelings? That's right, your heart! The heart brain is where we connect and communicate empathy, emotion, intention and values, relationships and compassion – both for ourselves and the world around us. When you are your feeling connected to your BIG, BOLD BEAUTIFUL life, you are connected to your heart brain.

Examples of how the heart brain communicates:
"I feel"
"I remember"
"I love", "I cherish", "I adore"
"I can relate"

The gut brain (enteric brain) or Enteric Nervous System (ENS) is two thin layers of more than 100 million neurotransmitters. They are connected through nerve cells that are in the lining of your gastrointestinal tract that flows from the oesophagus in your throat, all the way down to your rectum. The gut brain, also known as the "second brain", keeps information flowing through an intricate pathway of nerves that connect from the gut to your head brain, through the vagus nerve (which we will uncover the power of shortly). The gut brain influences emotional states of how you relate to the world around you. In fact, it is believed that up to 95% of serotonin (the happy hormone) is created within the gut, so it is also the seat of wellbeing, and feeling well. On an energetic level the gut brain is the "seat of the soul" – the home of your sense of self and your place in the world, of mission and purpose, knowledge, instinct, fear, intuition and identity. I like to think of the gut as the internal powerhouse, a central hub, where your intuition, curiosity and desire to live a BIG, BOLD, BEAUTIFUL life comes from. The gut brain is the starting point and connection point for all things BIG, BOLD, and BEAUTIFUL in your life.

Examples of how the gut brain communicates:
"I know"
"I can sense"
"I am feeling", "I am in my feels", "I have a feeling"
"I am"

TAPPING INTO THE THREE BRAINS TO CREATE IN ALIGNMENT TO YOUR BIG, BOLD, BEAUTIFUL VISION

Let's explore what's at play with the three brains when it comes to connecting and creating in alignment to your BIG, BOLD, BEAUTIFUL vision and taking action on your soul goals:

Your **head brain** wants to know that things are going to work out. It wants a good old pros and cons list and a spreadsheet. It demands logic, so it wants to know how it's going to happen, when it's going to happen and that it is going to happen. It's looking for examples, evidence and outcomes and hard and fast proof and assurances that it will all work out, otherwise it's not on board. No wonder there's so much over-thinking and going "round in circles" that can happen before you can take action!

Your **heart brain**, ah, the heart … it loves the dream, the vision of your BIG, BOLD, BEAUTIFUL life. It can feel it, it can relate to it, it can create all the beautiful pictures and scenarios of your BIG, BOLD, BEAUTIFUL life. With heart-eyed emoji vibes you feel the passion, the colours, the vibrancy, the romance, the dream, the beauty of it all. Your head wants it all, and it wants it now! The energy of the heart brain will keep you motivated even when the head brain is trying to take you off in a tailspin of decisions and getting in the detail of the "how" to make that beautiful, romantic vision a reality.

Your **gut brain** senses. It just knows. The gut works on instinct and intuition, which the head brain might find intangible ... because, where's the data to back it up, buddy? You will know when you are connected to the gut brain because no matter what your head brain is telling you, it makes sense to you; somehow, you know it will work out. Your gut brain loves to team up with the heart brain to create those fizzy, tingling, butterfly feels of excitement and possibility. When it's connected to the head brain with all that logic and over-thinking, you will rumble with a sense of caution, or even danger. And sometimes, when it comes to stepping out of your comfort zone on to the BIG, BOLD, BEAUTIFUL path, you will feel *all* the feels, usually all at the same time!

It's important to say that not one brain is more or less important than the others. You can't make decisions and take action based solely on emotions and no reason, in the same way that you can't just rely on logic and ignore your gut feelings. So, it's all about creating a dialogue, communication and the ability to connect to all three in a way that creates a new and dynamic way of supporting your BIG, BOLD, BEAUTIFUL journey. But it does require focus and awareness, as much as it requires dedication and practice.

That's why the BIG, BOLD, BEAUTIFUL journey is one for life, not just until the end of this book!

Here's a simple three-brain exercise to build the signal and communication muscles between the three brains:

EXERCISE

YOUR THREE BRAINS

Grab your journal or notebook and let's explore putting the three-brain concept into action. Start by taking an element of your BIG, BOLD, BEAUTIFUL vision, or a soul goal that you might be getting stuck on. Or that you might want to move forward with. And let's put it through the three-brain communication filter.

Remember to allow yourself to be curious and open. There's no right or wrong answer with anything you will explore, it's simply an opportunity to gain deeper awareness of how you communicate with yourself.

1. Let's start with your head brain.

- Bring your element of your BIG, BOLD, BEAUTIFUL vision, or soul goal to mind.
- Activate awareness in your mind (remove emotion and intuition for this part of the exercise); remember, this is the rational, objective, evidence-based brain.
- Think about the decision or choice you are making. Answer the following with regards to it …

Now explore the following questions in your journal or notepad, reflecting from your head brain.

- What are the facts around this element of your vision or goal?
- What are the pros and cons of bringing this element of your vision or goal to life?
- What will stay the same if you don't take this step or action?
- What will change if you do take this step or action?
- What's the best possible outcome from taking this step or action?

- What could be an unsatisfactory outcome as a result of taking this step or action?

Well done! Now take a breath and move on to your heart brain.

2. Drop your awareness to your heart brain.

- Breathe big and put your hand on your heart. It's time to move from logic and reasoning to emotion. Tune in and feel what's in front of you. Remember, this is the feeling, emotional brain.
- Slow down and take notice of the subtle cue of your heartbeat slowing or increasing.

Explore the following questions in your journal or notepad, reflecting from your heart brain.

- What is my heart telling me about taking this step or action?
- What does my heart want me to know about taking this step or action?
- What is the kindest and most compassionate thing I can do for me and my BIG, BOLD, BEAUTIFUL life right now?
- What incredible thing could happen if I were to follow my heart?
- What incredible thing wouldn't happen if I didn't follow my heart?
- How will my life be richer if I take action on this next step?
- What will I regret if I don't take this action on this next step, or any other step?

Lovely! Now take a breath and move on to your gut brain.

3. Gain awareness from your gut brain.

- Move your hand down to your belly, and breathe deeply into this area of your body. You should be able to push your hand out with your inhale and feel it retracting with the exhale.

As the gut brain is about intuition and instinct, you bring a curiosity beyond the logical to tune into what your gut might be telling you on a sensory level.

- You may find yourself saying, "I don't know." You might get a feeling rather than a clear thought. Don't judge it, don't try and rationalize it; simply breathe and allow whatever comes through to come through, however weird or wonderful it might seem!

Now explore the following questions in your journal or notepad, reflecting from your gut brain.

- What am I feeling about both the rational and the emotional aspects of this next step or action?
- What is my gut telling me about this next step or action? *This may be a sense of something rather than a clear thought. Explore what comes up.*
- What feels instinctual?
- What's important to me about this next step or action?
- How does this align with my sense of purpose?
- What feels best for my wellbeing right now?
- What is the compromise between my head and my heart that feels good to me right now?

Well done! You've just been on a connection quest between your three brains! Take a pause and take a breath.

4. Journal on your findings.

Once you've been through all three brain filters look back at your answers and journal on what you've explored to create alignment and connection to all brains for the next stage, or step on your BIG, BOLD, BEAUTIFUL journey.

My head brain needs …

Example: "My head brain needs a little more detail around this next step, so I will go back to my action plan, and make sure I've covered what's needed to feel confident about the way forward."

My heart brain needs …

Example: "My heart brain needs to feel the aliveness of what I am taking action on, so I will spend some time meditating on my vision map and connecting to how magical it feels."

My gut brain needs …

Example: "My gut brain needs to feel that the next step is aligned to my values, so I will check in to my energy and notice where I feel a 'push/pull' of energy."

When all three of them are working together my next step or action will be …

Example: "I will take some time to make sure I have a little more detail, and connect back into my vision and values, while also making sure I take some time to rest and dream about where this action is taking me."

Now that you've explored the three brains' needs and how they can communicate with each other for a clear sense of working together, you can create more of a dialogue between them when you are working on your BIG, BOLD, BEAUTIFUL soul goals.

Now let's dive deeper into what's going on with your inner landscape by travelling on the super-highway of connection of your vagus nerve to activate wellbeing and lines of communication throughout your body for ease of travel for your BIG, BOLD, BEAUTIFUL soul goals.

THE SUPER-HIGHWAY CONNECTION OF THE VAGUS NERVE, AND HOW IT CAN HELP YOU

Communication, communication, communication – it's such a vibe and a theme when it comes to living and creating your BIG, BOLD, BEAUTIFUL life in alignment with your vision map and soul goals. Most of the time when you're doing anything other than living it up BIG, BOLD, BEAUTIFUL style, it's because you're out of whack with your sense of self, or you're on a speed dial to fear and ego, and they're the ones calling all the shots.

But when you are in communication with your body's wisdom that's when you get to be in true connection with what is true for you on your BIG, BOLD, BEAUTIFUL path, as you take action. As you've already been exploring in this step, communication is happening all the time between your brain centres in the body, but how do they talk to each other, and what impact does that have on you grooving along with your BBB plans, or not?

You might think this is where it gets a little woo and otherworldly, and the inner workings of your body and mind are so in depth that you need a neuroscience, psychology and philosophy PHD to understand their full workings. Even then, there's so much that even science can't define when it comes to the connection of just what "consciousness" is, and how that connects through the conscious and unconscious parts of us as humans. I definitely believe there's a sprinkle of magic in there, but if you want to get down to the facts of what's going on in the wisdom of your body, your three brains – and all of your internal organs and your central nervous system – communicate through an extremely non-woo part of your autonomic nervous system called the vagus nerve.

The vagus nerve, also known as vagal nerve – vagus means "wandering" in Latin – is the main nerve of your parasympathetic nervous system that literally wanders from the brain stem to the gut, connecting to your major vital organs. As a core communicator it traverses both left and right sides of the body, and up and down – relaying sensory signals both from the gut and organs *to* the brain, and *from* the brain. As a core component of your parasympathetic nervous system (responsible for your fight or flight, or rest and digest states of being), your vagus nerve is signalling to your body at all times whether it feels safe to be and take action, or literally run for the hills. It's important to know this when you're working with your BIG, BOLD, BEAUTIFUL goals and micro-actions; if your body isn't feeling safe, it's going to be incredibly difficult to take steps and actions moving forward.

WORKING WITH YOUR VAGUS NERVE

What I find really fascinating (and where I get my body wisdom geek out on) is that we tend to believe that information flows from the brain and down to the body – that we think something, then feel it. Say you're thinking about your BIG, BOLD, BEAUTIFUL journey and you then feel overtly anxious or fearful about it, you might see that as a clue that either you can't do it, or there's something wrong with either it, or you. This can stop you from taking action.

Whereas what's actually occurring is that only 20% of information flows from the head brain down and the majority of information (80%) is coming from the gut brain through the vagus nerve via your heart and the rest of your major organs, collecting information along the way and sending it on up to the head brain where it processes that information into logical thought. So, your overall thought process and perception of any given moment is influenced by all three brains – starting with that sensing gut brain – connecting and communicating through the vagus nerve. This is why your health and wellbeing, along with vagus nerve regulation is so important.

I have found this particular field of study and information so incredible and useful to know when it comes to the BIG, BOLD,

BEAUTIFUL journey, because when you are as focused on your wellbeing and powering yourself up with self-empowerment – which you will explore in STEPS FIVE and SIX – you can work to reprogramme and create empowered thought patterns.

Being well means your mind and body will support your BIG, BOLD, BEAUTIFUL journey.

I think of the vagus nerve as the body's natural superpower, sending those supportive and useful communication signals to the places they need to go, to empower you on your BIG, BOLD, BEAUTIFUL journey. So, it's important to stimulate and maintain healthy function of your vagus nerve.

Here's some simple ways to do just that.

EXERCISE

SIX WAYS TO STIMULATE YOUR VAGUS NERVE

1. **Big Belly Breaths**

   Abdominal breathing is the key to activating the vagus nerve. Try out these simple breathing techniques:

   - Practise deep, slow belly breathing. Try and aim for six breaths per minute.
   - Place your hands on your belly and push out your hands with your breath. Expand your ribcage as you inhale. Bring your breath right back on the exhale to feel your hands sinking toward the back of your spine.
   - Exhale for longer than you inhale as this will trigger the parasympathetic relaxation response.

2. **Get the body moving ... gently**

   Practise embodiment exercises that activate the parasympathetic nervous system. These can help with digestion and blood flow, and include some gentle yoga, Yoga Nidra, tai chi and shaking. (More on that last one, shortly!)

3. **Sing it back**

   Singing, humming, chanting and gargling all activate the vagus nerve as it is connected to your vocal cords and the muscles at the back of your throat.

4. **Cold water**

   Yes, cold water really is a great stimulus for the vagus nerve. If a full body cold water immersion isn't quite your thing, then you can simply splash cold water on your face for a similar effect.

5. **Eat for gut health**

   - It kind of goes without saying that looking after your gut health is important when you consider that 80% of information is going from the gut and travelling up through the vagus nerve.
   - Adding good quality pre and probiotics, B12 and anti-inflammatory foods to your diet, will help support the vagus nerve.

6. **Spend time in nature**

   - Getting grounded and connected to nature is a sure-fire way to activate the parasympathetic nervous system and bring the vagus nerve into regulation.
   - You could:

     Spend time with the trees.

     Feel your feet on the earth.

     Stare up at the sky.

     Float in the still waters of a river, or the sea on a calm day.

Ongoing vagus nerve regulation is a simple yet powerful energy hygiene activity that will support you as you put the BIG, the BOLD and the BEAUTIFUL into what you are doing. It should play a fundamental part in activating your energy as well as maintaining your wellbeing for your BIG, BOLD, BEAUTIFUL life, and make working on your actions and soul goals so much better off!

Now that we've explored what's going on within the wisdom of the body, let's explore some of the magic that happens when you work with your energy!

THE POWER OF #ALREADYDONE

As you've discovered so far in this step you can do all the thinking, create all the plans, lay out the blueprints and all of the strategies when it comes to taking your BIG, BOLD, BEAUTIFUL vision and soul goals on the road ... But without tuning into the body wisdom and connecting from that seat of the soul – your intuition and the gut – you can only go so far before you start over-rationalizing, creating the kind of friction between the thinking, doing and being that creates a limitation to your BIG, BOLD, BEAUTIFUL plans – and causes all kinds of resistance, and mental chatter that keeps you stuck.

Getting stuck in worrying about "how" you are going to make your BIG, BOLD, BEAUTIFUL life a reality of the thinking head brain keeps all of the magic contained. It means that all the delicious possibilities of unexplored wild wisdom and wonder get locked up in a restrictive box. Your mind will play to a certain level, and then you might find that you can't bust beyond it, even when you've tried all the resistance-busting tools you explored in STEP THREE.

But fear not, because this is where you call on that "something more", which aligns the strategic (the practical) with the spiritual (the magic) to create the kind of expansive and elevated energy that provides the resources for your momentum on the BIG, BOLD, BEAUTIFUL journey.

The truth is that the BIG, BOLD, BEAUTIFUL journey doesn't make sense all of the time. It requires a huge amount of trust and surrendering to the process. It also needs your curiosity and willingness to look beyond any of the old habits and narratives that could keep you from not taking BIG, BOLD, BEAUTIFUL action. And it requires a commitment to seeing and doing things differently. Allowing yourself to lean in and explore beyond your current perception of reality means possibilities open up to you, and for you. You can connect to the energy of limitless possibility, and become infinite in your energy when you allow yourself to be open to the energy of the idea that anything is possible. This energy is where people often say they feel connected to the energy of the universe – something spiritual – something more.

Connecting to that "something more" allow you to explore beyond your current reality. It's where intuition, curiosity and the extraordinary love to play. It's the sense that there is something greater than you, something beyond the physical that can be connected with. I like to think of it as a connection of the intelligence of all the energy in the universe (and beyond), and the universe of energy you have within you. Like the acorn that has all the wisdom of a mighty oak tree inside of it, all the intelligence, energy and capacity you could ever need to bring your BIG, BOLD, BEAUTIFUL life existed the moment you created your BIG, BOLD, BEAUTIFUL vision.

It's this concept of the wisdom of the mighty oak that is already within the tiny acorn – the seed – that aligns to the concept that when you set your BIG, BOLD, BEAUTIFUL soul goals and vision map, what you are planting has all the wisdom within it to bloom into being. And that the moment you connect to it and write it down on your vision map, what you have planted is, in fact, #alreadydone.

And, to take this theory and concept even further, that what is #alreadydone in the BIG, BOLD, BEAUTIFUL vision you have created, and BIG, BOLD, BEAUTIFUL life you are creating, has an energetic vibration to it. Your BIG, BOLD, BEAUTIFUL vision and life will operate at a higher vibrational frequency than – say your everyday to-do list or life without purpose – so when you are in alignment, and matching to, the higher energetic vibration of your BIG, BOLD, BEAUTIFUL vision and life, you become intrinsically connected to the higher frequency of energetic vibration that creates it. Energetic magic in action!

EXERCISE

CREATE AN EMBODIED EXPERIENCE VISUALIZATION

Let's explore playing with the energy of the body's wisdom, the energy of #alreadydone, and being a vibrational match for your BIG, BOLD, BEAUTIFUL vision and life, with a simple embodied visualization exercise.

To create an energetic vibration frequency within you that matches with the energetic vibration frequency of your BIG, BOLD, BEAUTIFUL vision and life, close your eyes, take some deep centring inhales and exhales and allow these prompts to wash over you.

Connect with what you become aware of, and your sensory experience (your feels). Don't judge any of it, just notice. There's no way you can do it wrong, so allow yourself to get curious. If you find your mind wandering, or getting chatty, simply take some breaths and reconnect back in. If it gets too chatty, you may want to come back to the exercise another time when you feel able to relax into it. There's no rush.

Let's explore:

- Connect back to the BIG, BOLD, BEAUTIFUL vision of your life you created in STEP ONE.
- See it, hear it and feel it, as if it were right here with you in the present moment.
- Visualize and daydream that what you desire for your BIG, BOLD, BEAUTIFUL life already exists right here in the present moment. It is #alreadydone. Any actions now, or at any point moving forward, are simply proof points that you are showing up for it.
- How does the inevitability of the fact that it is #alreadydone feel in your body?
- Allow it to fire up and fizz inside of you, and then settle and be with you.
- What sensations or feelings do you notice? Where do you feel it in your body?
- Are the feelings moving or still? If they move, how do they move? In which direction? Are they fast or slow?
- Just notice what you notice.
- Can you see any pictures, or imagery? If you can, are the images moving or still? Are they in front of you? How big? Are they in a frame or panoramic? Are you part of the picture itself or on the outside looking in?
- What colours can you connect to? How bright are they? How clear?
- If you can hear sounds, what sounds can you hear? How close or far away are these sounds? Are they clear or muffled? Which direction is the sound coming from?
- Now, let's dial up that energetic frequency within your body to become a vibrational match for the BIG, BOLD, BEAUTIFUL energy of what you are connecting to.

- Take a deep inhale and exhale.
- Imagine you have a dial in front of you. You can move the dial, to turn up the feelings and sensations until they feel like they are vibrating in every cell of your body.
- Breathe big.
- If the image you see is in front of you, imagine moving toward it so you can climb into it, become part of the image, make it into a movie that you are part of. In your mind's eye, dial up the intensity of the colours and clarity; make them more vivid and bright.
- If the sounds that you heard sounded distant, bring them closer to you or move toward the sounds, turn up the volume, make it so that you can hear it all clearly.
- Dial up all of the energy on what you feel, see, hear and connect to with the energy of #alreadydone.
- Continue to inhale and exhale, deeply and gently, for two or three minutes or until this feels complete.

Well done! You have just created an incredible burst of energy in the universe and your body as you explore the vibrational match of your vision to your body. It's powerful stuff!

To share a beautiful story of where this magic came to life, I offered up this practice with one of the Kickstart your BIG, BOLD, BEAUTIFUL groups. My wonderful client Sarah shared her embodied vision with us. In it, she was sitting by a campfire at a cliffside on the rugged landscape of Western Portugal, with her campervan behind her. In her sensory experience she could feel the warmth of the fire on her skin, the glow bouncing from the people gathered around the fire. She could smell the smoke on her clothes that was evidence of travel, adventure and an enormous sense of freedom. As she looked around within her vision she saw she was in a circle around the fire with strangers who already had a deep connection to her heart. The conversations were life-affirming. While she was there on a travel adventure there was also an element of her being there to share her purpose of helping people through holistic health practices.

When she shared her epic adventure with us she spoke with such detail and knowing. Her whole energy had shifted. There was no doubt that this was #alreadydone. It's important to share that this was so far from Sarah's reality at the time. She worked in a hugely demanding job as a social work manager and she certainly didn't own a campervan!

But the seeds had been planted. Within the space of a year, Sarah had retrained as an holistic health coach, mind-body practitioner and Practical Magic coach. She had moved on from her social work job to start her purpose-led business. Before this new venture there was something else she needed to do. And after becoming the proud owner of a T@B 320 caravan, Sarah set off on an epic three-month, 4,600 mile solo adventure through France, Spain and Portugal. Not once did she question her decisions, because it was #alreadydone, and who was she to push back on what she had anchored into the energetic experience she had created?

It doesn't mean you have to give up your job and pack up your life for an epic solo adventure (unless that's what you truly desire). But an embodied experience visualization is your opportunity to dial up the energetic vibration of your BIG, BOLD, BEAUTIFUL vision and life. It helps you to bring it into the present and imprint the energy of inevitability of #alreadydone onto your physical and sensory experience.

Now you have explored the energetic experience of #alreadydone, let's take this a little deeper, with some deeper embodiment and practical application.

THE ENERGETIC ELEVATION OF YOUR BIG, BOLD, BEAUTIFUL LIFE

Your body knows exactly how it feels when you have all of the incredible gifts that are in your BIG, BOLD, BEAUTIFUL life and, as you have just explored, you can become a vibrational match for it.

As your body feels it, and anchors that feeling, all those juicy, wonderful signals get carried around by the wandering vagus nerve to tell the rest of you that you are readdddyyy. When you feel ready, you think ready, and then you're so ready to take BIG, BOLD, BEAUTIFUL action.

You can take it to the next level through something called "Energetic Modelling".

I first came across "modelling" as a concept within Neuro Linguistic Programming practices. Modelling is a practice in NLP that simply means "finding the structure of excellence". It is the process of creating – or modelling – the excellence that is your BIG, BOLD, BEAUTIFUL life through thinking, feeling, and the way you behave in accordance with it, through the lens of all that is BIG, BOLD and BEAUTIFUL. Then you can take this to an even BIGger, BOLDer, more BEAUTIFUL level, as you become the vibrational match to what is #alreadydone, by creating the energetic containers for your BIG, BOLD, BEAUTIFUL life. So that the way you speak, act and behave creates an energetic, physical and somatic manifestation of your BIG, BOLD, BEAUTIFUL vision to create an anchor point between the the energetic and the physical.

What does this mean in practice? Well, say one of the elements of your BIG, BOLD, BEAUTIFUL vision is that in order to become known in your field of purpose and excellence you are out there sharing your voice and your work. As part of your BIG, BOLD, BEAUTIFUL vision you are a magnetic and powerful public speaker. You don't just like it, you love it. You are in your absolute element when you are doing it. You are so good at it, in fact, that you are invited to speak on stages and at key events wherever in the world you want to be. And you get paid well to share your expertise.

In order to be that vibrational match, you have to know and feel what it's like to be rocking it from that stage, even if you've never done it before! In other words, how you speak, think, feel and act in every moment from hereon in, gets to be in alignment with the energy of the BIG, BOLD, BEAUTIFUL vision and life you have created.

That may feel like somewhat of a stretch right now but what if I were to tell you that you can achieve and receive all the excellence you need from someone else who has it in abundance by modelling how they do it? Curious? Let's explore.

THE WAY YOU THINK

The way you think in accordance with your BIG, BOLD, BEAUTIFUL vision and soul goals really has the most profound impact. The more you can *think* in accordance with the vibrational match of what's within your BIG, BOLD, BEAUTIFUL vision, the more your head brain will create the blueprints and neural pathways that take you to it. This is more than thinking, thinking, thinking until you have steam coming out of your ears, or having a positive mental attitude – it's about building the mental and emotional resilience that will support the journey.

Thinking strategies that will support your BIG, BOLD, BEAUTIFUL journey include:

- Having a beginner's mindset
- Cultivating a growth mindset
- Adopting curiosity and creativity as part of the natural process
- Building mental and emotional resilience
- Failing forward (as explored in STEP THREE)
- Looking after your mental, emotional, physical and spiritual wellbeing (much more of this to come in STEP SIX)

- Connecting regularly to your BIG, BOLD, BEAUTIFUL vision
- Getting practical and strategic support
- Modelling - adopting or "borrowing" the empowering thought processes of successful people (more of this in the next chapter)

THE WAY YOU SPEAK

Changing up how you talk to yourself, and how you communicate with the world around you, can often mean changing the narrative that might keep you stuck. Because the words you speak to yourself, and to the world, matter. Your internal dialogue and external dialogue create your reality. Words have power. The words you speak show your perception of your world around you, and that shapes your beliefs, and drives your behaviour in alignment to your BIG, BOLD, BEAUTIFUL vision.

Here's some simple yet effective ways your language and self-talk can support your journey:

- By removing apologetic language – anything where you are using "just", "small", "little". For example, talking about your "little" business, or "just this thing" you're working on. What you are doing is important to you. Talk about it like it's important. Adjust your language by owning your energetic power. Think, "My creative business", or "An important project" you're working on.
- By changing from "have to", "need to", "should" (which are all based in fear, obligation and conformity). Instead, switch to, "I get to" and "I am" (which are rooted in choice, ownership, presence and action).
- By using curiosity language: changing from "that's weird" or "that's strange" to, "I'm curious to find out more about this," or "I'm looking forward to discovering what this all means".

Can you feel the difference, in shifting from disempowering to empowering language? It's a simple yet incredibly powerful and dynamic shift that will make a huge difference as you navigate your BIG, BOLD, BEAUTIFUL journey and life.

It's important to get curious, so that you can gain awareness of the words, phrases and language patterns you use that may not serve you. Think about what you could change them for to support your BIG, BOLD, BEAUTIFUL journey.

Have a play in your journal, in two columns:

Disempowering language:	Changed to empowering language:
Example: "I'm not sure this is ever going to work; whenever I've tried anything like this before I've failed miserably."	*Example: "I am open to how this unfolds. I can take learning from previous experiences to help support the success of what I'm doing this time around."*

THE WAY YOU ACT AND BEHAVE

The way that you act and behave supports your BIG, BOLD, BEAUTIFUL vision and goals. You can act and behave in positive alignment with what you are creating, or you can act out of alignment. You can take action, or you can procrastinate. You can – and will – behave in ways that support what you are working toward, or you can – and will – behave in ways that can disrupt your progress.

Some of it will be conscious – you will be aware you are procrastinating by cleaning your entire house rather than working on your action points. And some of it will be unconscious – you may not be aware that your behaviours are hindering your BIG, BOLD, BEAUTIFUL progress. You might be working really hard on a project, then stopping before its completion because you're unconsciously afraid of how successful it might be. Or you could take on another project at work in a job you don't want to be in, because unconsciously it will mean any spare physical or thinking time will be taken up, rather than working on your BIG, BOLD, BEAUTIFUL soul goals.

Your conscious behaviours can be easier to deal with. Your *unconscious* behaviours can be sneakier, and more difficult to understand what's at play. The most important thing is gaining awareness of what your empowering and disempowering behaviours are … because you can then do something about them.

Acting and behaving in alignment with your BIG, BOLD, BEAUTIFUL vision and soul goals means they are inevitable because you are working on them, and with them. These behaviours show up as:

- Taking ownership of your goals and vision
- Taking action, even micro-actions
- Seeking support and getting accountability to ensure you stick to your goals and planned actions
- Looking after and nurturing your wellbeing
- Taking space and time as you need to
- Creating healthy emotional and energetic boundaries (which we will explore more in STEP FIVE)
- Spending time in inspiring environments, surrounded by like-minded people who will support your growth
- Adopting physiological, energetic body language in alignment with your BIG, BOLD, BEAUTIFUL self in your BIG, BOLD, BEAUTIFUL life, e.g. holding yourself in your physical and energetic energy of being in alignment with your BIG, BOLD, BEAUTIFUL vision and life

Allow yourself – with compassion – to get real and reflect on what actions and behaviours could be holding you back and how you can put things in place to create actions and behaviours that support you instead. For example, "I make myself busy doing things that take up all of my time, even though I don't *have* to do them. Doing them mean I don't have the time and space to focus, or take action, on the BIG, BOLD, BEAUTIFUL vision I desire."

EXERCISE

ENERGETIC MODELLING

Now, let's take all of what you've just learned, and try this energetic modelling exercise to super-charge how you speak, think, feel, act and behave in alignment with your BIG, BOLD, BEAUTIFUL life.

You are going to explore modelling the behaviour of someone you admire for their BIG, BOLD, BEAUTIFUL approach to life by taking notice of how they do it, and you are going to try it on for size yourself. Then you can adopt this good stuff, and wear it like the finest outfit around town!

When you are carrying out this energetic modelling exercise, you can either work with someone you know – a role model, mentor, work colleague, family member or friend – where you can sit down and ask them questions about their thought and feelings processes. Make sure you share with them why you are doing it. Alternatively, you can simply observe, as it may be someone you may not have direct access to, such as a role model or famous person you have long admired. Your "model" can be alive or dead; it's their energy you are connecting into. Take some time to observe and journal through the following questions:

- Who is this person?
- What are they known for?

- Why do you admire them? What is it about them that you admire?
- Notice their behavioural patterns – the ways in which they might think, feel, speak, act and behave – that you admire. How do they seem to achieve their results? What do they do that is different to someone else who might not get the same results as them? How do they go for what they want?
- How do they carry or hold themselves? What is their body language like? How do they walk into a room? How do they greet people?
- What are some of the powerful words or phrases they use? What is their empowering self-talk? What do you think they might say to themselves to help them feel confident? How do they talk to themselves when they have had a setback? (You can imagine this if you don't have direct contact.)
- How do they interact with people? How do they get the best out of people? How do they honour their boundaries? How do they delegate effectively? What are some of their empowering leadership skills?
- What support and guidance do they call in? Spiritual, emotional, mental or physical?
- How do they accept compliments or praise? How do they deal with rejection? How do they deal with feedback? How do they give feedback?
- How do they deal with conflict? How do they manage themselves in a crisis? What do they think, say, behave and feel?
- How does this person nurture and look after themselves? How do they honour their time? What is their self-care routine? What do they do to relax? What are their wellbeing routines for their mental, emotional, physical and spiritual wellbeing?

Now that you've observed the way they think, speak, feel and behave when they are being their BIG, BOLD, BEAUTIFUL selves, you are going to try on some of their energetic magic on yourself.

Find somewhere quiet, breathe big, and bring forward in your heart and mind a scenario where you would like to be working at a level of excellence in your BIG, BOLD, BEAUTIFUL vision. For example, speaking confidently in front of people, being in an interview for your dream job, or taking a BIG, BOLD, BEAUTIFUL action toward one of your soul goals.

Now, you are going to adopt some of the traits, actions and energy of your "model".

- Breathe deeply into your abdomen and belly.
- Bring the imagined scenario into your mind and body.
- Picture your "model" playing out in the scenario, and then imagine floating into their body, so that you can try everything you are exploring on for size.
- Replay the movie in your mind and body of them doing what they do in the way they do it. See what they see, hear what they hear, and feel what they feel, as they are carrying out their behaviours and actions in the movie you are playing of them in your dream scenario.
- Now, float back into your own body, bringing with you all the learnings that are useful for you to use both now and whenever you need them.
- Replay the movie in your mind and body, with you as the main protagonist – speaking, thinking, feeling, acting and behaving armed with all of the good stuff you explored from your "model".
- Keep breathing deeply into your abdomen and belly.
- Feel what you feel, see what you see, hear what you hear as you are doing your thing.

- Do this a couple of times, playing the movie in your mind and body until you feel comfortable with your performance.
- Break out of this state by doing something mundane like thinking about the colour of your front door, or what the weather is doing right now.
- Continue with whatever you want to do.
- Find a space to practise these new energetic skills you've adopted as your own.
- Keep coming back to this exercise. Practise trying on your new energetic skills and attributes for size to connect to how bloody great it feels to have them inside of you.

You will find that the more you connect with this energetic and embodied modelling practice, the more it becomes something that is part of you. This practice is also a great vagus nerve activator as firing up your physiological state sends juicy energy signals between the gut-heart-head axis – dynamic physical "states of being" lead to dynamic thinking "states of being".

Finally, it's great to explore this exercise to model different empowering attributes you admire or require, from different people, so you can get what you need from a variety of energetic sources you admire. It's like an energetic embodiment pick and mix!

Now, imagine taking all of this juicy mind-body and energetic wisdom and taking it to the next level through activating the energy of joy. Oh yes, we are going there ... let's go!

ACTIVATING THE POWER OF JOY TO DIAL UP YOUR BIG, BOLD, BEAUTIFUL ENERGY

"The fact is always obvious much too late, but the most singular difference between happiness and joy is that happiness is a solid and joy a liquid."

J.D. Salinger

So, you've explored an incredible amount to dial up your energy and connect into the infinite wisdom and wonder of your body ... but we haven't yet explored perhaps the most fundamental part of what gives energy to the BIG, BOLD, BEAUTIFUL journey, and that is JOY!

I've never met or worked with anyone on this BIG, BOLD, BEAUTIFUL path who doesn't want a joyful life. I mean, just check in with yourself and your vision for a moment. Is there any part of your BIG, BOLD, BEAUTIFUL vision that doesn't feel joyful to you? If not, I would suggest heading back to STEP ONE and sprinkling that vision and those soul goals with a healthy dose of joy; it's an energetic activator and force.

Joy is a sure-fire way to create energetic elevation to put the pep in your step for your BIG, BOLD, BEAUTIFUL vision and soul goals. For me, seeking joy over happiness is much more sustainable because it is something created from within – you can feel joy as a way of being in existence with your BIG, BOLD, BEAUTIFUL life.

Joy is the rich inner world of personal growth – the freedom, the values, the inspiration, the relationships, the spiritual and creative expansion of being in your BIG, BOLD, BEAUTIFUL life. Whereas happiness is the moments of this joy that exist in the outer rewards: the holidays, the home, the job, and the things you have as a result of doing within your BIG, BOLD, BEAUTIFUL life.

To truly *live* your BIG, BOLD, BEAUTIFUL life is the embodiment of joy as an energy. It's also a simple super-power that becomes the energetic current of your BIG, BOLD, BEAUTIFUL journey. It is the wind beneath your BIG, BOLD, BEAUTIFUL wings.

Some of the powerful impacts of joy as an energy elevation are:

- Joy is a way of being – a way to live, rather than a fleeting state. It is inner contentment, fulfilment, satisfaction. It doesn't rely on external drivers.
- Joy is a powerful energy activator. It brings you the energy you need to get things done and it will give you energy when you need it most.
- Joy will keep you going. It will sustain you over a long period of time, because you are working with and toward it, as an internal driver and a positive state of being.
- Joy is a fundamental part of wellbeing. Both happiness and joy are great for activating the parasympathetic nervous system. It lowers your heart rate, reduces stress and boosts your immune system.
- Joy is found in simple pleasures. It can be everywhere you look for it: in the laughter of friendship, the majestic power of nature, and in the powerful energy of being present and in connection with your BIG, BOLD, BEAUTIFUL life.

The most powerful way I have discovered to activate joy as an important part of the BIG, BOLD, BEAUTIFUL fuel for the journey, is firstly to recognize and remember that joy is a fundamental part of why I am choosing a BIG, BOLD, BEAUTIFUL path. Without joy, what would be the point, right?

And then, secondly, I choose to bring joy into the journey by being disruptive with it. This is a great one to not only bust beyond resistance and to create some BIG, BOLD, BEAUTIFUL energy and momentum, but to also disrupt you from doing the same things you've always done, which could have been holding you back until now. You will also find that joyful ways of doing, being and creating become so much more rewarding.

One of the things we do halfway through the Kickstart Your BIG, BOLD, BEAUTIFUL Life Programme, is a seven-day challenge to disrupt your ego from wanting to crawl back under the comfort zone blanket, and to stop the brain trying to go back to habitual patterns.

Want to explore this for yourself? Give the Seven-Day Disruptive Joy Challenge a go.

SEVEN-DAY DISRUPTIVE JOY CHALLENGE

Carry out the joy challenge, and keep a diary or journal your findings at the end of each day. Remember to stay open and curious as you explore and reflect on the different challenges each day. You can even share the challenge with a group of friends so you share your experiences, and be motivated by each other's joy amplification!

Day One

Your first disruption challenge is to do something different to your everyday, which is going to bring joy into your day and into the day of others. Do something unexpected for a colleague, friend, partner, housemate or family member or send love energetically to everyone you come across throughout your day.

Examples: Compliment a stranger, tell someone something you admire about them, share with a colleague, friend or loved one what they did for you that had a positive impact on your day/week.

Journal on your joyful reflections at the end of day one.

Day Two

Reach out to someone you've never spoken to before, or someone you come into regular contact with but don't often engage with, to find out about something that makes them feel joyful.

Journal on your end of day two reflections – What did you find out? What are your joyful reflections?

Day Three

Today, you are going to learn something completely new.

- This could be a new word, a new fact, or something that's going to expand your knowledge in relation to your BIG, BOLD, BEAUTIFUL vision.
- It could be something you've learned from a friend, your partner, your kids, your colleagues. It could be something about your cat / dog / hamster / goldfish, which you didn't know before today.

Journal on your end of day three reflections – What new fact did you learn? What are your joyful reflections about this?

Day Four

Today, you are going to do some form of exercise you've never done before, even if it's for five minutes. This could be a new exercise, a new class, a new movement practice, you name it. Maybe you'd like to try dancing or hula hooping – something, anything, that is going to get your body moving!

Journal on your end of day four reflections – What new exercise or movement practice did you do? What are your joyful reflections?

Day Five

Today is about disrupting negative thought patterns that come in throughout the day. When you catch them you are going to disrupt them with a counter-joy disruptor.

For example, if someone is majorly peeing you off – again – instead of going down the usual route of "Why do they always do this?", disrupt the thought with something joyful instead.

Or, if you're bagging on yourself, what could be the counter joy-disruptor to your inner critic?

Journal on your end of day five reflections – How were you your very own kindness ambassador? What are your joyful reflections on this?

Day Six

Today's joyful disruption challenge is going to take you to new places. It's time to go somewhere in your local area that you've never been before. This could be to a new building, a park, a street, finding a blue plaque, or another place of historical or environmental importance in your local area.

Happy discovering.

Journal on your end of day six reflections – What new discovery did you make? What are your joyful reflections?

Day Seven

And here you are on the last day of the Seven-Day Disruptive Joy Challenge.

The last challenge today is super simple. You're going to find a different route to the one you would normally take.

This could be your route to work (if you go out to work), the route you take on a daily walk, or a different way home. Anything.

On this different route you are going to take notice of something joyful that catches your eye.

Once you have completed your seven-days of disruptive joy take some time to reflect on the week. Journal on the following questions:

- What did you notice about activating the power of joy throughout the week?
- How will joy help to support your energy and motivate you for your BIG, BOLD, BEAUTIFUL journey?
- What will you continue to do to bring joy into each day and on each step of your BIG, BOLD, BEAUTIFUL journey?
- How will you commit to your own joy?

Now that you've experienced the simple yet powerful energy activator of joy, this is just the beginning. You can come back to this exercise, any time you would like a joy top-up.

Remember that joy is your birthright. You deserve it, you are it, you have the power to create it, and it will be the heartbeat that carries vital energy to all areas of your BIG, BOLD, BEAUTIFUL life. It will provide a wellbeing wellspring to help activate your parasympathetic nervous system, and fire up embodied joy energy up your vagus to your head brain. Full vagus joy, baby!

BIG, BOLD, BEAUTIFUL JOY!

STEP FOUR REVIEW TIME

Wow! What a journey of discovery and energy activation we've been on in STEP FOUR. It's been deep, and it's been rewarding. This step is a powerful one to come back to when you are wanting to get in energy alignment with the BIG, BOLD, BEAUTIFUL soul goals and vision you are creating, and any time you need an energetic boost. Here's a checklist of the exercises and activities to help you put more power to your potential:

✓ Use the *Three Brain Exercise* to communicate more effectively with head, heart and gut intelligence for a more balanced approach to working on your BIG, BOLD, BEAUTIFUL soul goals.
✓ Use the techniques to activate the super-highway connectors of the *vagus nerve,* in co-regulation with your nervous system and wellbeing, that ultimately supports you as you take action on your BIG, BOLD, BEAUTIFUL journey.
✓ Activate the *energetic power of #alreadydone* with the powerful visualization exercise. Use it to create a *vibrational match* for your BIG, BOLD, BEAUTIFUL vision, and anchor an embodied physical and sensory imprint, to make that vision an inevitability.
✓ *Embody your energetic elevation* with an energetic modelling technique. Allow it to empower and support the way you speak, think, feel, act and behave as you take action on your BIG, BOLD, BEAUTIFUL journey.
✓ And finally, activate the *all-important super-power of JOY* as the energetic current of your BIG, BOLD, BEAUTIFUL life, with the Seven-Day Disruptive Joy Challenge.

Now that you've embodied your expansion, and explored dialling your energy up, it's time to groove on over to STEP FIVE. Let's keep it all going, by creating a self-empowerment toolkit that will serve and support us in all areas of our BIG, BOLD, BEAUTIFUL life.

But before you dash over to STEP FIVE, enjoy a BIG, BOLD, BEAUTIFUL Breakout Ritual, which will activate your body wisdom and power up the embodiment magnificence you've explored in STEP FOUR.

BREAKOUT RITUAL
MOVEMENT ENERGY ACTIVATOR

I learned about creating movement rituals from Rochelle Schieck, founder of Qoya. They are a great way to honour the energy of different touchpoints in your life, or the passing of one phase of life into another through movement, and the energy in motion through your body. This is great when you are working with your soul goals. It's a way of honouring your transition out of your past (what you are leaving behind), your present (and all the incredible resources you already have) and what you are bringing into your future (through your BIG, BOLD, BEAUTIFUL vision).

To create your movement ritual, get clear on what it is you would like to work with. This might be one element from your vision map, or one of the key areas on that map that you would like to energetically focus on, such as love, self-love, abundance or creativity.

Ask yourself, what do I want to honour with my movement?

You are going to create a movement with your body that signifies past, present and future.

MOVEMENT ONE: RELEASING THE PAST

Create a movement with your body, based on the past, or what you are leaving in the past.

Consider:

- What you are letting go of, or what you have already let go of. (This could follow on from the release rituals at the end of STEP THREE.)
- Release anything that doesn't serve you.
- How does this feel in your body?
- What movement would signify this? (I find shaking it out works really well for me.)

- Find some music that would work well. I love something up tempo, so that I can shake out / release what I am letting go of, but this could be something gentle and flowing for you.
- Breathe deeply and let your body move with the movement to signify release.
- Continue the movement until the song has ended.

MOVEMENT TWO: GIVING THANKS IN THE PRESENT

Create a movement based on the present and all the resources you already have available to you.

Consider:
- What inner skills and resources you already have.
- What you have already achieved.
- What are you grateful for?
- How does this feel in your body?
- Create a simple movement that relates to how you feel about everything that is already present.
- Find some music that would work well for this movement. It could be something really uplifting and upbeat, or slower and deeply meaningful.
- Breathe deeply and let your body move with the movement that signifies your present.
- Continue the movement until the song has ended.

MOVEMENT THREE: EMPOWERING YOUR FUTURE

Create a movement based on your BIG, BOLD, BEAUTIFUL vision and what you are calling in.

Consider:
- What you are calling in.
- How you will move in alignment to your vision of the future.
- Your gratitude for everything you have created.

- How powerful do you feel in this vision of the future?
- How does this feel in your body?
- Create a simple movement that signifies your vision of the future and everything you are creating in your BIG, BOLD, BEAUTIFUL life.
- Find some music that aligns with your vision of the future. I find something empowering and uplifting works really well.
- Breathe deeply and let your body move with the movement that signifies your present.
- Continue the movement until the song has ended.

Once you have your three movements and songs, you can dance your movement ritual anytime you would like, to embody the energy of release, gratitude and empowerment.

This is also really good as a daily movement practice. It shouldn't take any longer than 9–15 minutes.

STEP FIVE

CREATE A SELF-EMPOWERMENT TOOLKIT

"When we spend our lives waiting until we're perfect or bulletproof before we walk into the arena, we ultimately sacrifice relationships and opportunities that may not be recoverable, we squander our precious time, and we turn our backs on our gifts, those unique contributions that only we can make."
BRENÉ BROWN, *DARING GREATLY*

In this voyage of discovery on the path to your BIG, BOLD, BEAUTIFUL life you've explored ways in which you can stay true to your BIG, BOLD, BEAUTIFUL vision. You've revealed how you can carve your own path by getting focused and taking action with your BIG, BOLD, BEAUTIFUL soul goals, and how to move beyond resistance and dial up your energy, to keep the momentum and fire alive within you.

All great stuff and so ripe for the BIG, BOLD, BEAUTIFUL quest. Wouldn't it be great if that were all of it? But alas, not just yet. The number one thing I see time and again, that will hold most people back from thriving in their vision and desires, is the lack of self-belief about the capabilities and skills they have to be able to take continued and aligned action on their BIG, BOLD, BEAUTIFUL soul goals.

All too often they give up. Or they may not have even made it this far, because the inner voice telling them it's not possible becomes louder than the inner cheer squad keeping them going.

Creating and living this BIG, BOLD, BEAUTIFUL life means stepping up and showing up for it – no matter what might come your way while you are making it happen. The process is one of learning, shifting, shaping and growing. Growth is not linear. Your journey will have many plot twists and turns, ebbs and flows, and ups and downs, but everything you are learning here will be your guide.

If you are feeling all the feels and questioning yourself and your ability, and yet you are still here reading this, then I want you to give yourself a big high five. Because being willing to show up, and being curious enough to be open to the idea of seeing and doing things differently, takes courage. The truth of it is, that a lot of people won't have got this far.

And instead of getting stuck in the doom scroll – wishing you had the confidence and motivation to do half the things that you see others doing, or beating yourself up for not having the guts to do the things you really want to do, and wondering if you ever will – you are here, and you're doing it. I applaud you because I know how much it takes.

So, let's take that and delve into STEP FIVE on this epic journey of your BIG, BOLD, BEAUTIFUL life, because BOLD is the word! In this step, you will explore ways to fire up your self-belief by creating a self-empowerment toolkit full-to-bursting with techniques that you can dive into every time you need a power-up, for each and every stage of this BIG, BOLD, BEAUTIFUL adventure.

Everything you are going to create within this self-empowerment toolkit supports your BIG, BOLD, BEAUTIFUL vision and soul goals, as well as being BIG, BOLD, BEAUTIFUL empowerment tools for life.

IN STEP FIVE YOU WILL:

✓ Explore your beliefs, and how they can be either the fuel or the foe on your BIG, BOLD, BEAUTIFUL mission as you move forward with your soul goals ... and how to create the kind of *rocking self-belief* that will have you cooking on gas from this point forward.

✓ Uncover ways to *become an unapologetic badass*. Flip the script on your apology behaviours and show up fearlessly for your BIG, BOLD, BEAUTIFUL vision.

✓ Learn all about the *positive benefits of compliments*, and why they are not just nice to haves, but good for mind, body, brain and soul.

✓ Learn why "NO" is a complete sentence and why exercising your NO muscles creates *healthy boundaries* – the perfect containers within which to cultivate your soul goals and bring your BIG, BOLD, BEAUTIFUL vision into blooming being.

✓ Create the fertile conditions for your BIG, BOLD, BEAUTIFUL soul goals by *watering the seeds of change* rather than getting bogged down by doubt.

✓ Discover the importance of spending time in places, spaces and with people who will help you elevate and collaborate as you take action, and activate even more JOY into your BIG, BOLD, BEAUTIFUL life. Get ready to *gather your soul crew!*

CREATING YOUR ROCKING SELF-BELIEF

Living and creating from your BIG, BOLD, BEAUTIFUL life really comes down to believing in yourself and your ability to make it happen. And that self-belief is something unique to each and every one of us. There may be some areas of your life where you feel you can rock out with your socks out and others where you will wobble all over the place.

While it would be amazing to wave a wand and have all the self-belief and confidence you feel you need to conquer the world – believing in yourself and your abilities is not something that happens overnight. It's not like you wake up one day free from those doubts and fears that have been holding you back. BUT there is a way through.

The secret sauce for creating rocking self-belief begins with being curious enough to challenge your limiting thought patterns and habits. And then it's about being flexible and curious enough to try out and adopt some new ways of thinking, acting and behaving, in alignment with your BIG, BOLD, BEAUTIFUL vision. The idea is to make it a high-kicking, high-flying reality and feel good doing it.

As you've already witnessed throughout this book – awareness is key to creating action – so let's start creating your rocking self-belief by getting an awareness of your belief system. We need to look at how it might be holding you back right now, and what you need to support your BIG, BOLD, BEAUTIFUL vision and goals instead. This is about flipping the script on limiting or disempowering beliefs to transform them into the kind of rocking beliefs that are going to be the rocket-fuel for your BIG, BOLD, BEAUTIFUL journey.

WHAT IS A BELIEF?

Simply put, a belief is a state, or habit of the mind, where you accept something to be your truth regardless of whether you have the evidence to back it up. For example, someone can hold a belief that the Earth is flat, regardless of evidence supporting the fact that the Earth is round. In the same way, you can hold a belief that you are not capable of seeing something through, despite evidence that you see countless things through to the end on a daily basis.

Your beliefs are your set of filters for how you view the world and your place within it. You hold beliefs about the external world, e.g., what goes on around you, and you hold beliefs about your internal world, e.g., how you think, feel, act and behave in accordance to the world around you. They act like sets of internal commands based on your perception of what is happening around you at any given moment in time.

Your beliefs are the brain's (and body's) way of making sense of an often confusing and complex world. They form the guiding principles that provide direction and meaning, becoming what is known as your model of the world.

Your own personal belief system – and your model of the world – gets created from a young age. In fact, psychologists believe that by the age of seven, you have taken on board all of the 'information' to form your belief systems, habits and behaviours that can set you up for life. These are created based on experiences you've had, the stories of the world you grew up around, the morals and guiding principles of significant people you have in your life as you grow up, the culture and community you have been part of, the teachings you had at school, as well as the media that your parents or guardians consumed. All of these shape the narratives and guiding principles you grew up around and mostly live by now. So much so, that you may not be consciously aware of all that are at play (some of them you will be). Many create unconscious behaviours and habits related to those beliefs systems and principles we were a part of in those pivotal years.

For example, think about your relationship to money – what are some of the phrases you might use, or have heard when you were growing up? "Money doesn't grow on trees." (This was a classic in our house, although I can still picture a tree growing cash in my mind's eye in an instant!), "Money doesn't buy happiness." "As long as you work hard, you will always have money." All of these phrases easily roll off the tongue, and drip drip drip into your unconscious mind to form your belief patterns around how difficult money might be to attain, enjoy or your relationship to hard work.

The challenges you will navigate as you step out of your comfort zones toward your BIG, BOLD, BEAUTIFUL vision mean you will be required to bust beyond some of the old belief systems you hold about yourself and your model of the world. And some of these old belief systems are going to be at odds with what you desire for your BIG, BOLD, BEAUTIFUL life. They hold fast because they have not been challenged … until now.

So, if a limiting belief is simply something you accept as the truth, or a story you tell yourself, could it also be possible to believe that you can take an empowering belief and put that in the place of a limiting belief? And that new shiny empowering belief can then become something you accept into your life and being as a new truth?

What if you could create a new model of the world that puts the fuel to the fire of your BIG, BOLD, BEAUTIFUL instead?

Exciting right? Let's try it out.

EXERCISE

FLIP THE SCRIPT ON YOUR BELIEFS

Let's explore flipping the script on your limiting beliefs by turning them into empowering ones. Grab a notepad or journal, and on the left-hand side of the page write out all of the limiting beliefs you have about yourself. This is anything that could hold you back from living your BIG, BOLD, BEAUTIFUL life. Then, on the right-hand side, create a counter-belief that forms an empowering belief.

LIMITING BELIEF	EMPOWERING BELIEF
Example: "I am rubbish at relationships. I always pick the wrong person and it ends in disaster."	Example: "I have learned some key lessons from relationships that have gone before. And I have discovered what works for me, and what doesn't. I am ready, willing and capable of showing up for myself as part of a healthy and committed relationship."

Come back to this exercise any time you find yourself doubting yourself and your abilities. Get curious about what the beliefs are that you hold (whether conscious or unconscious), explore them, and then flip them! Those doubts are simply limiting beliefs you hold about yourself, and as you've discovered above, you get to rewrite them to find empowering beliefs that will help support you from hereon in.

BECOME AN UNAPOLOGETIC BADASS

Now that you've explored the idea of limiting to empowering beliefs, it's time to take it to the next level through playing with your language and behaviours. As you discovered in STEP FOUR, the way you think, speak and act create your reality. Your words have power. Creating an empowered external dialogue can create an empowered internal dialogue; in other words, what you give voice to can create a physiological response. Take this as an example: if you were to say, "Getting on a stage and speaking in front of 1,000 people? I could never do that!" How do you think your body would respond to what you've said? Not well, right? I mean it's highly unlikely you would feel confident enough to get out and rock that mic!

On the flip side, one of the most powerful ways to dial up your confidence and create self-empowerment (and dial up the energy in your BIG, BOLD, BEAUTIFUL life) is dial up your outer language and dial down on how apologetic you are in the way you speak, act and behave. These apology habits show up *everywhere*. They are a marker for how you feel about yourself and your abilities.

They show up in how you express who you are to the world (think about what you wear, or what you are too afraid to wear, but would love to), they show up in the way you interact with the world – from the way you interact with a group of people, how you speak up (or don't) in a discussion or debate, to how you ask for support (or again, don't), even down to how you start and close a conversation, or begin and sign off an email – your apology habits show up pretty much everywhere.

These apology habits – specifically over-apologizing – are the ultimate buzzkill when it comes to your BIG, BOLD, BEAUTIFUL journey, because you are communicating to the world that you are too small for the magic you are creating. The more you apologize for yourself, the more you're telling the world around you – and most importantly, yourself – that you don't think you're up to the task of living it BIG, BOLD, BEAUTIFUL style. Over-apologizing will keep you playing small. It will keep you hidden, and it sends out the message that you're not worth the things you desire most for you and your BIG, BOLD, BEAUTIFUL life.

Again, like beliefs (because habits are formed from beliefs), your apology habits can often be so ingrained they are unconscious. You may be subconsciously seeking reassurance from others, or working from internal limiting beliefs, so it's important to bring out those apologetic habits into the light of day so you can see them for what they are. That way, you can change the narrative and behaviours that are holding you back from creating BIG, BOLD, BEAUTIFUL momentum.

GET TO KNOW YOUR APOLOGY BEHAVIOURS

You know you're over-apologizing if you:

- Over-justify your opinions or why you're upset about something
- Over-explain yourself
- Caveat everything
- Apologize for showing emotion
- Constantly put yourself down or belittle yourself
- Talk about how boring your problems must be
- Start most of your sentences with the word, "Sorry"
- Say "sorry" when there's no need
- Use apologetic language. For example, "Sorry I couldn't get back to you sooner ..."; "I'm sure you already know this ..."; "I'll be really quick. I know you must be busy ..."

Once you start becoming consciously aware of your apologetic behaviours they can't go unnoticed. And when you gain that beautiful awareness of where they are showing up you can start working with them to create empowering habits out of them instead. It takes a bit of time to unravel that automatic apology reflex, but the more you do it, the more powered up you start to feel ... and the more resilience you build for when things don't go according to plan too.

So, let's try this on for size, and start the break up of all break ups ... with your apology habits!

EXERCISE

EMPOWER YOURSELF BY BREAKING UP WITH YOUR APOLOGY HABITS

Taking some of the apology behaviours you've just explored, start taking notice of your own apology habits. Use this exercise to get curious about where they come up for you most. Then, turn those disempowering apology habits into empowering unapologetic badassary!

Here are some of my own examples:

My apology habit is ...
Over-using the word "sorry".

My unapologetic habit will become ...
Swapping "sorry" for "thank you". So, "Thank you for bearing with me while I learn more about this"; "Thank you for receiving me as I am."

My apology habit is ...
Starting emails / conversations at work with, "I know you must be busy," or "I hope you don't mind me disturbing you."

My unapologetic habit will become ...
Recognizing my worth by removing apologetic phrases in all places and spaces where I communicate at work.

My apology habit is ...
Saying, "Does that make sense?" every time I share something.

My unapologetic habit will become ...

Making it active, rather than passive, by changing my language: "What questions do you have?" or "What are your reflection points on what I've just shared?"

Now it's your turn to go through your apology habits on the left and then counter them with the unapologetic habits you could create on the right.

Apology habit: Unapologetic habit:

....

....

....

Apology habit: Unapologetic habit:

....

....

....

Apology habit: Unapologetic habit:

....

....

....

Apology habit: Unapologetic habit:

....

....

....

Now that you've broken up with your apology habits, filtering out some of the negative narratives, it's time to take this to the next level by actually receiving in the good stuff to support all that is BIG, BOLD and BEAUTIFUL ...

COMPLIMENTS PLEASE

It's all too easy to push away the nice things people say to you because of those pesky old beliefs and narratives we've explored in this step so far. You may be familiar with the ones that say, "You mustn't be too big for your boots," or the one that is playing on the eternal loop of "just who do you think you are?" if you were to say or believe something good about yourself.

But the truth is that by not allowing internal or external praise or celebration in, an unconscious habit is formed to build an emotional wall to the point where it becomes a hundred times harder to accept praise than it does to accept criticism.

For example, if someone were to say something nice to you, and someone else were to say something critical, which are you more likely to listen to and believe? The compliment or the criticism? It's an unfortunate fact that most of us would think a compliment as an untruth, and accept a criticism as a fact. The challenge this creates for the BIG, BOLD, BEAUTIFUL path is that the more we refuse to accept good things in, the harder it becomes to take notice when your soul goals are weaving magic into your life.

Why do we do struggle to accept compliments? Well, there's a number at things at play – from issues with self-esteem, to feeling cognitive dissonance, through to being a trauma survivor – all of these things can disrupt your ability to accept compliments, or accept criticism over praise. But at a core level, it's most likely that it comes back to the concept of negative bias, which has been so important for our survival. We have evolved based on becoming wise to negative situations. We even have a dedicated region of the brain (the amygdala), which is designed to translate and respond to fearful and stressful situations, so we can learn from them. The faster you learn from a negative situation, the better your chances of survival.

In the world we now live in, that thinking no longer aids us as it did. Having a negative focus – rather than harnessing and celebrating what you're good at – won't create the conditions you need to bring your BIG, BOLD, BEAUTIFUL vision wholeheartedly to life. So, it's time to get working on gaining that all-important awareness and reprogramming the things that don't support the BIG, BOLD, BEAUTIFUL journey to let the good stuff in!

Yes, it's time to get down with compliments. And it goes something like this:

"I love that dress you're wearing."

"What, this old thing? I got this in a charity shop years ago. It's got holes under the armpits … look!"

Ahem … Let's try that again …

"I love that dress you're wearing."

"Thank you. I really appreciate you saying that; it's made my day."

Notice the difference?

Compliments are the gift that keep giving. They provide external indication and evidence of things shifting to the BIG, BOLD, BEAUTIFUL life, and you can use them to start embodying and connecting to how empowering that feels in your body.

Compliments are good for:

Confidence

Motivation

Happiness

Performance

Self-compassion

Resilience

Interpersonal relationships

Increased wellbeing

Your connection to what you are
creating

Gratitude

Science backs up that it's good for our brains to be told that we're good at something; from the feel-good dopamine reward hit, to building neuroplasticity, through to improving motor skills, and increasing focus and energy. And through compliments you can recognize your own good stuff to help empower yourself on your BIG, BOLD, BEAUTIFUL journey. It's something that you can come back to time and again when you need a confidence power boost.

Accepting compliments is easier said than done, so let's explore the three keys to accepting a compliment:

1. *Receive and pause.* When you receive a compliment, check your automatic response – wait three seconds before consciously responding.
2. *Acknowledge.* Practise saying, "Thank you."
3. *Reflect.* Praise the compliment, "Thank you. That means a lot to me."

With these three simple steps you can become a compliment-receiving pro. And to bring compliment receiving into practice – and power up your self-empowerment good stuff – use the following exercise to track compliments.

SELF-EMPOWERMENT TOOL

CREATE A COMPLIMENT TRACKER

Start using this compliment tracker on a daily basis to power up your self-empowerment as you take action toward your BIG, BOLD, BEAUTIFUL soul goals. At the end of each day, journal on the compliments you received. Write them out and reflect on each one.

- What was the compliment regarding?
- How did you respond to it?
- How does it make you feel?
- Where do you feel that compliment in your body?
- What can you do to remind yourself of it when you most need it?

Keep your compliment tracker to hand so you can delve into things that keep coming up, or patterns you notice that you can learn about yourself as a result. Use it any time you need a power boost, or to remind yourself of your good stuff.

Now that you've explored how to bring the power of compliments into your life, it's time to create the conditions that are going to keep this BIG, BOLD, BEAUTIFUL show on the road. Yes, it's time to explore your boundaries!

NO IS A COMPLETE SENTENCE: ESTABLISHING HEALTHY BOUNDARIES

"When you say 'yes' to others, make sure you're
not saying 'no' to yourself."
PAULO COELHO

One of the best ways you can say more "YES!" in your BIG, BOLD, BEAUTIFUL life is by learning to say a whole lot of "NO!" to others. You guessed it; I am talking about boundaries.

OK, so we all have a desire to be seen, loved and accepted, so saying no to people when you would normally be bending over backwards may seem like one of the biggest hurdles you are going to face on this quest for a BIG, BOLD, BEAUTIFUL life. But believe me when I say that this is one of the most powerful tools you will ever have in your self-empowerment toolkit. Discovering and honouring your boundaries is a tool for life that will protect your energy, and preserve and nourish your joy.

This is where you begin the journey to ditching your people pleaser tendencies and the over-bearing weight of feeling responsible for everyone else's happiness (an impossible task, BTW).

Creating healthy boundaries ensures you have the best conditions possible for your BIG, BOLD, BEAUTIFUL soul goals to take shape. It puts the BIG, the BOLD and the BEAUTIFUL in your life. So, we are going to explore boundary setting in depth in this section, along with a number of exercises to help you compassionately create and strengthen boundaries where you need them.

WHAT ARE BOUNDARIES?

Boundaries are the invisible lines that communicate how you allow others to treat you and where your own personal thresholds are in relation to your feelings, your needs, your responsibilities, communications and physical space. They are intrinsically linked to your core values (as you discovered way back in STEP ONE).

If your core values are the guiding set of principles, or the markers in the road of your BIG, BOLD, BEAUTIFUL journey, then your boundaries are the barriers that keep you from careering off the road and into the ditch!

That's may seem a little dramatic I know, but it's important for you to know where you are likely to give most of your energy away to others by not having your boundaries in place, because that will distract you from what you are focusing on when it comes to taking action on your BIG, BOLD, BEAUTIFUL soul goals. Instead, creating healthy boundaries will help you leverage toward your BIG, BOLD, BEAUTIFUL vision.

Your boundaries are not for other people; they are for you. Basically, they are the bouncers on the door of your BIG, BOLD, BEAUTIFUL life. You may not be aware of what your boundaries are, but you will know they're being crossed when you notice feeling resentful or pissed off. Knowing how you feel when you have leaky boundaries is a useful starting point, as you can follow the feeling to show you how they affect you, and then take action.

TYPES OF BOUNDARIES
Physical

This includes your physical space – your home, your office, your bedroom. You will know if your physical boundaries are being over-stepped if:

- Someone repeatedly comes into your physical space without asking, or continually doesn't respect your physical space.
- They might look through your drawers or cupboards.
- They might make a mess in your home, move things around, break things or borrow without asking.

Personal

This is your own space. Your level of comfort in your personal space can be different to someone else's. You will know when your boundaries are being over-stepped when:

- Someone gets too close to you physically, or "invades your personal space".
- You don't feel comfortable with being touched, hugged or kissed.
- Your identity is not respected.

- How you express yourself by what you wear, or your appearance, is constantly commented on.

Emotional & Energetic

This can be difficult to quantify, but you definitely feel it. You will notice:

- Feeling heavy around a friend or family member who often unloads their problems to you. You have to really gee yourself up to see them.
- Carrying the emotional load of those around you.
- Constantly trying to "fix" or make things better for them.
- Feeling exhausted around some situations or people, or in certain environments.
- Feeling drained of all your energy.
- Things seeming one-sided – so, you do a lot of the emotional labour in a relationship or situation, and it's not reciprocated.
- Not feeling supported about the things that are really important to you.

Time

There's nothing more precious than your time, so if you don't ever feel you have enough hours in the day, it will be down to time boundaries. Over-stepping of time boundaries could look like:

- Being asked to work longer hours as an expectation or sign of commitment to your work.
- Being contacted by your boss when you're on holiday when you've made it clear that it's not OK for them to do that.
- Being expected to work over-time without appropriate recompense.
- Being asked to do something when you have expressed how much you already have on.
- Being left waiting by someone who's never on time.

Intellectual

Your personal viewpoints, intelligence and perspective are yours, and they should be respected. You'll know when someone is over-stepping an intellectual boundary when:

- You've been told you are being stupid for having a difference of opinion.
- Your opinions or passions are disregarded, ridiculed or disrespected.
- You feel you are talked over, shouted down or condescended to.
- Your qualifications, experience or education have been belittled or are not merited.
- You've made it clear that you don't want to engage in a debate and the other person pushes on regardless.

Material

Your material possessions and belongings, which also includes financial boundaries. This could be your home, your car, your clothing or anything that you own. This could show up as:

- Someone borrowing something from you and bringing it back broken (or not returning it at all).
- Being guilted into lending money (whether or not it gets paid back).
- Withholding money that is owed or has been promised.

Wellbeing

This relates to honouring the things you need to keep you feeling well and healthy. It might include nutrition, exercise, sleep, alcohol, even medication. When your boundaries are over-stepped, this could show up as:

- Not respecting your choice to not take alcohol or drugs and pressuring you to do so.
- Being made to feel guilty about resting or exercising.
- Disturbing rest and exercise time.
- Not supporting you with healthy eating or nutrition by either disregarding your diet choices or tempting you with unhealthy choices.

When it comes to working on your BIG, BOLD, BEAUTIFUL soul goals, pretty much all of these boundary areas will influence your ability to focus and achieve them. But the ones that have the biggest impact tend to be around time, energy and emotional support.

But I share this now – this is going to require a whole lot of self-compassion, practice and commitment, because the people pleaser within you is not used to saying no. You will have to deal with the anxieties, worries and guilt of feeling like you're letting people down. You may tell yourself you're selfish for wanting what you want, which may seem to come at the price of doing and being everything for everyone else. And let's face it – there are going to be some people in your life that do quite well out of your leaky boundaries, so they might struggle when you start asserting your new boundaries because they may not benefit them.

You might already be noticing where your boundaries are being respected or disregarded, or where you haven't established them yet. You may be acutely aware of the impact this has on your sense of self and your energy levels. It's so important to understand how poor or leaking boundaries affect you, so that you can do something about it. And it's only you that can do that.

As always, it starts with awareness. So, before we move on to explore a number of exercises that can help you establish and maintain healthy boundaries, let's review where yours are, or are not, right now.

EXERCISE

LEAKY VS. HEALTHY BOUNDARIES

Make a note below each type of boundary to explore leaky boundaries that cause issues for you vs. healthy boundaries that will support you. This will help you gain awareness before you take conscious action to change things up.

Here's an example to get you started:

Physical leaky boundaries example:
"My in-laws pop around at any time of the day or evening without checking that it's OK for them to do so. It's never a quick visit, and often disrupts what I am working on. I feel I have to entertain them."

Physical healthy boundaries example:
"My bedroom is my space for relaxation and wellbeing. It's a space where I can really unwind and feel at peace. I keep it tidy and clean. My partner respects this by picking up their clothes from the floor and tidying up after themselves."

Explore what leaky and healthy boundaries are for you through each boundary type:

Physical:
Leaky boundaries are ...

....

....

Healthy boundaries are ...

....

....

Personal:

Leaky boundaries are …

....

....

Healthy boundaries are …

....

....

Emotional & energetic:

Leaky boundaries are …

....

....

Healthy boundaries are …

....

....

Time:

Leaky boundaries are …

....

....

Healthy boundaries are …

....

....

Intellectual:

Leaky boundaries are …

....

....

Healthy boundaries are …

....

....

Material:
Leaky boundaries are …

....

....

Healthy boundaries are …

....

....

Wellbeing:
Leaky boundaries are …

....

....

Healthy boundaries are …

....

....

Now that you've started exploring the principles of leaky and healthy boundaries, take the learning into the next set of exercises, to establish, create and maintain boundaries that are going to empower and support you to achieve your BIG, BOLD, BEAUTIFUL soul goals and vision.

SELF-EMPOWERMENT TOOL

ESTABLISHING, CREATING AND MAINTAINING HEALTHY BOUNDARIES

There are seven key ingredients for establishing, creating and maintaining healthy boundaries that will help you on your BIG, BOLD, BEAUTIFUL vision and soul goals journey and for a BIG, BOLD, BEAUTIFUL life. They are:

Attention

Awareness

Acknowledgement

Compromise

Communication

Commitment

Self-compassion

The idea is that you can use some of these mini exercises to help you get from awareness to conscious action and change things up.

ATTENTION

Tune in to any of the leaky boundaries you just explored (physical, personal, emotional, etc.) and pay attention to where and how you are feeling in relation to them. As you are already aware, your body will communicate when things are out of alignment.

Consider:

- Where and when you feel emotionally and physically exhausted.
- What your gut feeling is about what's going on.
- Where you feel frustration or resentment. Is there tension in your head, shoulders, neck, gut or back? This often indicates that you are carrying more than your fair share.

What are you noticing in your energy and your body in relation to certain people, places and environments, scenarios or situations in relation to your leaky boundary?

ATTENTION example:
"When my in-laws visit, without checking whether it's a good time for them to do so, I can feel myself getting increasingly annoyed. I notice this as a rising feeling of tension in my chest that moves up to my shoulders. I find myself feeling frustrated, as well as anxious that I am not able to complete what I was working on. All the time they are here I am thinking about what I'm not able to do. I find myself being quite snappy and short with them, and thinking unkind thoughts about how they are imposing on my time and space, which then makes me feel bad."

Now try paying close attention to one of your leaky boundaries and explore how it makes you feel:

....

....

....

AWARENESS

Your values are your inner drivers for your BIG, BOLD, BEAUTIFUL life, and your boundaries ensure that you keep to the path of the journey you're on with your vision and your soul goals. Gaining awareness of how your values show up through the filters of physical, personal, emotional, energetic, time, material, intellectual and wellbeing boundaries (as defined in TYPES OF BOUNDARIES, p. 167), means you can honour them and bring them into each aspect of your life, which can ultimately drive your behaviour.

AWARENESS example:

One of your core values is JOY. So, in your BIG, BOLD, BEAUTIFUL life, you honour your boundaries in order to maintain JOY in the following ways:

Physical: Your personal spaces (office, home, bedroom) – you have plants, crystals, photos of people you love, pictures that bring you joy.

Personal: You wear bright, bold, patterned clothes that make you feel joyful.

Emotional and Energetic: You are at your best when you are around people and within environments where you feel joyful and energized, rather than drained and uninspired; you search out those places.

Time: You carve out quality time to do things that bring you joy – whether this is with other people, or things you like to do on your own.

Material: Any personal affects you have that bring you joy are treated with respect. You have autonomy and money to spend on things – or experiences – that bring you joy.

Intellectual: What you find joyful is respected and supported, even if it's not 100% understood.

Wellbeing: You enjoy exercising and eating well. Feeling well makes you feel joyful and feeling joyful is a fundamental part of your wellbeing.

Use this AWARENESS to take your core values and put them through your boundaries filters to give you ideas as to how you can honour your values through creating healthy boundaries …

Reference back to your core values exercise on pp. 16–18. My core values are:

....

Put them through your boundaries filters:

Physical ....

....

Personal: ....

....

Emotional / Energetic: ....

....

Time: ....

....

Material: ....

....

Intellectual: ....

....

Wellbeing: ....

....

ACKNOWLEDGEMENT

Recognizing and acknowledging what you stand to gain by having your healthy boundaries in place helps you with making your BIG, BOLD, BEAUTIFUL vision a reality. Think of it like a mission statement that supports your BIG, BOLD, BEAUTIFUL life. Declare it! Double points if you share this with others so you can hear yourself claim it, or have it somewhere you can see it, to remind yourself often.

ACKNOWLEDGEMENT example:

"By having healthy boundaries in place, I am able to work on my BIG, BOLD, BEAUTIFUL soul goals, because I will have more time and energy. Honouring my boundaries makes this journey of discovery a more joyful experience, which is incredibly important to me."

Create your own declaration of what you stand to gain from having healthy boundaries in place:

....

....

....

COMPROMISE

It can be incredibly difficult to start saying "no", or asserting your boundaries straight away, especially to the biggest boundary pushers you have around you. That's especially the case when it comes to creating the time, space and energy you need to take action on your BIG, BOLD, BEAUTIFUL soul goals. There may be instances where you start gently, by finding a happy middle ground, but where – ultimately – you can still establish boundaries on your terms. This is where your soon-to-be-favourite phrase: "That doesn't work for me, but what I can do instead is …" will start coming into play.

COMPROMISE example:

"Could you stay a little later at work tonight so that we can run through this presentation ahead of tomorrow's meeting?"
Response: "Staying on this evening doesn't work for me. But if you let me see where you're up to now, I can give my feedback within the next hour, and we can schedule some time first thing tomorrow to make sure everything is in place."

... Notice what is willing to be done, what is not, and how there is no justification or apology in here too!

Now try it out yourself:

Take one of your leaky boundaries that could get in the way of taking action on some of your BIG, BOLD, BEAUTIFUL soul goals. Play with some ideas for compromise on your boundaries on your terms:

One of the biggest leaky boundaries that could impact on my progress toward my BIG, BOLD, BEAUTIFUL soul goals is:

....

....

....

What I'm not available for (what you are not willing to compromise on):

....

....

....

What I am available for (what a compromise could be instead):

....

....

....

Explore your compromises anytime you come across them, and they become second-nature.

COMMUNICATION

Communicating and reaffirming your boundaries is your responsibility. You cannot expect people to read your mind about your needs, or expect them to be in step with you when you change things if you don't make your boundaries clear. This may seem challenging to begin with, but it's so worth it. Keep it simple. Share why you're doing it, and how they can help support you (and NO apologizing!).

COMMUNICATION example:
"I will share my boundaries with those who they affect the most, such as my partner, my family and my work colleagues. I will sit down with each of them, tell them what I need, and why it's important for me. I will make it clear if there are things I can no longer do, or which might need to change, as a result of the BIG, BOLD, BEAUTIFUL plans I'm working on. We can find a way to collaborate so that both sides are happy."

Explore with whom you will communicate your boundaries and how you might do that:

....

....

....

COMMITMENT

Establishing and maintaining healthy boundaries takes work. You have to be willing to stay committed and persevere. You also have to be prepared to *assert, honour, defend and re-establish* your boundaries when they are tested or rough-roaded, which they will be!

Creating a plan for how to deal with scenarios when boundaries get blurred or crossed, or when you feel your boundaries are not being honoured, will help you get back on track.

COMMITMENT example:

You've agreed with your workplace that you can reduce your working days from five to four, because you desire a better work/life balance, and you would like to develop a creative project. This has been agreed and communicated clearly with your peers and clients, but online meetings creep into your diary or deadlines are not met, which means you have to complete work on your agreed day away from work anyway.

For this example ...

You *assert* your boundaries by:

- Negotiating priorities that mean that you may not be able to get a project / piece of work completed within your agreed hours, in which case it is given to someone else.
- Saying "no" firmly and without over-justifying yourself or apologizing – this takes practice.
- Having a clear out of office on your inbox and voicemail on your work phone, which make clear your working hours, and who to contact in case of an urgent enquiry.

You *honour* your boundaries by:

- Not reacting with anger or passive aggression, but remaining calm and re-establishing your boundaries and agreements made about them.
- Working with a mentor, or someone you admire, whose boundaries align with yours. Model their boundaries (you can use the energetic modelling exercise on p. 136).

- Explaining to others you work with why work/life balance is so important for everyone.

You *defend* your boundaries by:
- Standing by them and recommitting to them.
- Not giving in and doing the work – even if it is easy for you and will only take five minutes.
- Sticking to the routine you've established around them.

You *re-establish* your boundaries by:
- Recommunicating them as and when needed – to new team members, new clients, when there are new ways of working.
- Reinstating them if they lapse.
- Reminding yourself why they are important to you.
- Agreeing on – and setting – realistic expectations around what can be achieved within the time you have available for work.

Now, create some of your own boundaries COMMITMENT ideas:

I will assert my boundaries by:

....

....

I will honour my boundaries by:

....

....

I will defend my boundaries by:

....

....

I will re-establish my boundaries by:

....

....

As you did when *acknowledging* your boundaries, remind yourself of your commitments often, and keep coming back to them if you find your boundaries need reinforcing.

SELF-COMPASSION

Sometimes – and in certain situations – it will be easier to establish and maintain healthy boundaries. Other times, it's going to be tougher going. There are going to be times when you feel bad because you're not available in the ways you were before. You will feel guilty for putting boundaries in place if you think it means other people are negatively impacted as a consequence. And in some situations, you are going to have to deal with people who struggle as you establish and reinforce those boundaries.

This is where self-compassion, and being as kind to yourself as humanly possible, comes in. You will need to remind yourself – often – that it is not selfish to honour your boundaries and focus on your BIG, BOLD, BEAUTIFUL vision. And it helps to remember *why* you are putting these boundaries in place by connecting to your vision (which will so often have a positive impact on those around you anyway!). Yes, there are going to be a few people who will have to adjust, but this is their responsibility, as much as setting and honouring your boundaries is yours.

Ways in which you can practise self-compassion when establishing and maintaining healthy boundaries:

- Focus on your wellbeing.
- Give yourself permission to say "no".
- Be kind to yourself. The guilt may feel real at times, but you can work through it by being as compassionate with yourself as possible.
- Remind yourself why you are doing what you are doing – and why it's good for others, not just you.
- Ask for support from a therapist, mentor, coach or energetic running buddy.
- Create accountability for your BIG, BOLD BEAUTIFUL goals, and maintaining your boundaries.
- Give yourself some breathing space if you, or someone else, has tested your boundaries.
- Practise letting go of frustration and anger toward those who seem to want to constantly push your boundaries (this will only direct your energy to the wrong place).
- Focus on what you can control. Find ways to let go of the rest. Yes, it's a biggie, I know!

What other self-compassion ideas can you come up with?

....

....

....

As you are no doubt aware from working through these exercises, there's much to unpack when it comes to making sure you are supporting yourself in a way that helps you create the right kind of conditions for your BIG, BOLD, BEAUTIFUL vision and soul goals. Establishing and maintaining healthy boundaries is a lifelong commitment and approach to living your BIG, BOLD, BEAUTIFUL life, so keep coming back to these boundary exercises on a regular basis.

WHAT DO YOU STAND TO GAIN?

Creating conscious awareness of what you stand to gain is one of the key ingredients for sustaining and bringing into bloom all of the wonderful things you are creating for yourself and your BIG, BOLD, BEAUTIFUL life, and what has made it so worthwhile putting those healthy boundaries in place for!

It makes sure you are emotionally and energetically providing the right kind of conditions for those seeds you planted when you first formed your BIG, BOLD, BEAUTIFUL vision map (p. 27). This means that, rather than tending and giving energy to the weeds of doubt, you will water the seeds of BIG, BOLD, BEAUTIFUL change. My goodness, I do love a gardening metaphor!

Watering the seeds of change by forcing on what you stand to gain means lifting yourself up and out of the fear space you might find yourself in. It's about changing your focus from the "what ifs?" of doom, which focus on what you could lose, and instead focusing on "what if? wonders" of what you will bring into your BIG, BOLD, BEAUTIFUL life.

This is going to be an ongoing commitment to reframe and refocus, but believe me, it's so worth it. Head to the next exercise, and let's explore.

SELF-EMPOWERMENT TOOL

WATERING THE SEEDS OF CHANGE

Follow these four simple steps for committing to watering and tending what you stand to gain as a result of your BIG, BOLD, BEAUTIFUL vision and soul goals. Remember to practise self-compassion as you go through this awareness activation exercise.

1. Become aware when fear and anxiety are slipping into the "what ifs" disaster movie scenarios.
2. Reframe the "what if" disasters into "what if" wonders.

What if disasters:

Example: "When I share about how I really feel, and what I really want for my life, people are going to think I'm crazy/ greedy/too much and will leave me. I will be alone."

What if wonders:

Example: "As I grow and develop into my authentic self, some people may fall away. That's OK; they are not for me anymore. I will attract more people into my life who get me, and who I feel sustained, supported and nourished by."

....

....

....

....

....

3. List out as many scenarios that your fear or ego might be coming up with and change them up.

4. Recommit often to the changes you're making and the reasons for making them (your why – your BIG, BOLD, BEAUTIFUL vision and life).

Now that you've discovered so many incredible tools for your own self-empowerment, it's time to find your people who will help you on your BIG, BOLD, BEAUTIFUL journey … for life!

GATHER YOUR SOUL CREW

"If you want to go fast, go alone; if you want to go far,
go together."
AFRICAN PROVERB

What's next in your self-empowerment toolkit? The company you keep. I cannot tell you how important it is to be in the right kind of environment, and with the right people, to sustain your BIG, BOLD, BEAUTIFUL journey. Surrounding yourself with like-minded cheerleaders, champions and energetic running buddies, will mean that you always have someone holding your BIG, BOLD, BEAUTIFUL vision up for you to see when you've lost sight of it – which you will – and who will remind you of just how possible it is for you to get where you want to be.

It's time to gather your soul crew. They are the merry bunch of misfits and soulful rebels who will be there for the wobbles, will help you celebrate the wins, and will provide you with a supportive and non-judgemental space in which to be both vulnerable and BIG, BOLD and BEAUTIFUL. They will show you all the bloody incredible things about yourself that it's often so difficult for you to see, and will also show you the evidence that you are not in fact failing, you are making progress – even when you feel it's not happening fast enough. (Damn you, ego!)

They will also show you some of the biggest lessons you will learn, through their own experiences and BBB journey too.

So much of what you are exploring in this guide has come from the experiences of those who've been through the Kickstart Your BIG, BOLD, BEAUTIFUL Life Programme. There's a constant learning when people come together to explore more. The thing I love the most about the curious soul seekers who've embarked on the BBB journey, is the friendships and energetic bonds that are made because of the exploration and non-judgemental space held. Conversations are had that would never happen outside of these spaces.

Having a space where you can be seen, heard, felt, understood and get a true sense of belonging, is one of the most potent self-empowerment tools you can have for your BIG, BOLD, BEAUTIFUL life, so let's explore how you can start finding *your* people who will share the ride with you.

HOW TO FIND YOUR SOUL CREW

Explore these ideas, and then come up with your own:

- Try new things; be open and curious to exploring new ideas and places to go to explore them. Take what you need and leave the rest behind!
- Join a group programme or sign up for a course or retreat where there's a group/community element built in.
- Step out of your "woo" closet to find and attend events about things you are curious about.
- Spend time in places and with people who will help you elevate your energy, not drain it. If you're not into big groups or loud places, find somewhere with small groups of people, in a more intimate setting.
- Go to events, meet-ups or groups related to your interests. If it doesn't yet exist, start one up!

- Get to know people around you on a deeper level. Get curious – find out if you have shared interests or commonalities.
- Get involved in a community project; it's a great way to meet people who have shared interests and a common vision.
- Say yes more times than you say no! As easy as it can be to stay in your comfort zone, especially if you're an introvert, there's so much great stuff waiting for you. Practise saying yes 2 out of 3 times and see where your adventures take you.
- Get like-minded friends involved so you have a curious soul seekers friend date on a regular basis.

By gathering your soul crew, you will find yourself open to so much more than you ever could have thought possible. Believe me when I say that the reward in doing so will so BIG, BOLD and BEAUTIFUL, you will feel like the luckiest human alive!

STEP FIVE REVIEW TIME

STEP FIVE has been power-packed with so much impactful self-empowerment that will support your BIG, BOLD, BEAUTIFUL vision and soul goals. Come back often, and delve deeper into what's in this step, as you continue on your BIG, BOLD, BEAUTIFUL journey. Because believe me, what you have explored puts the power into self-empowerment.

Here's a checklist you can delve into as you progress on your BIG, BOLD, BEAUTIFUL journey:

✓ *Break up with your apology habits* to become a #sorrynotsorry unapologetic badass and create empowering habits to support and sustain your BIG, BOLD, BEAUTIFUL soul goals.

✓ Create a *compliments tracker* to help you connect to the BIG, BOLD, BEAUTIFUL in your life and get you a power-up boost from the inside out when you most need it.

✓ Delve into all of those juicy *healthy boundaries* exercises to create, communicate and cultivate the kind of positive and healthy boundaries that will support you in your BIG, BOLD, BEAUTIFUL soul goals, and life.

✓ Create the right conditions and *change the "what if" disasters into "what if" wonders* with the simple stepped approach.

✓ Explore ways to *gather your soul crew* so that you can spend time being with people, and in places and spaces, that will help elevate and empower your BIG, BOLD, BEAUTIFUL goals, the journey, and your life!

It's time to turn the page and progress to STEP SIX where you will master ways to nurture yourself and your BIG, BOLD, BEAUTIFUL life through self-care.

But before you dive into the next step, why not try the BIG, BOLD, BEAUTIFUL Breakout Ritual? Find your Crystal Power Squad, who will provide the energetic power vibes to support your self-empowerment good stuff!

BREAKOUT RITUAL
CREATE YOUR CRYSTAL POWER SQUAD

Crystals have powerful healing and energy activating properties. They are great for any kind of situation. Need to activate love energy? Rose quartz is a go-to. Need to clear or cleanse your space of negative energy? Clear quartz or selenite will do the job. Want to speak your truth? Wear some lapis lazuli around your neck.

There's literally a crystal for everything.

But which crystals create the kind of energy you need for confidence and powering yourself up from the inside out as you take action on your BIG, BOLD BEAUTIFUL soul goals?

I reached out to two of my go-to crystal experts and BIG, BOLD, BEAUTIFUL clients. Suzy Pike from Spike Rocks creates beautiful jewellery using crystals. Marie Andrew from Mother of the Spiritual Child uses crystals for energy healing and creating harmony at home.

Here's what they had to share on creating your own Crystal Power Squad for self empowerment.

SUZY'S CRYSTAL POWER SQUAD: CARNELIAN, BLACK ONYX AND PYRITE

Suzy says, "Carnelian is the absolute go-to for creating empowerment from the inside out. It keeps your feet on the ground and everything stable, while also lifting your vibes and keeping your energy high.

"Black onyx is the perfect stone for creating and maintaining healthy boundaries. Its protective energy keeps your hopes and dreams sacred while working like your own personal trainer to power those dreams' vibrancy and vitality.

"And then there's the one and only pyrite. Pyrite packs a golden power punch to put fire to your inner fuel. And while it's the ultimate energy protector, it's also the ultimate empowerment activator. It's basically like having your very own cheer squad when you wear it.

"Wearing, or holding, a combination of carnelian, black onyx and pyrite – especially around your heart or solar plexus – will give you all the power and protection you need to turn your goals into empowered action."

MARIE'S CRYSTAL POWER SQUAD: CARNELIAN, TOURMALINE AND TIGER'S EYE

"Carnelian is a significant stone when it comes to creating courage, self-belief and confidence. It's always the stone I will place at the centre of a crystal grid as the central, activating energy to give power to the rest of the grid and create an energy activation space at home.

"Tourmaline is the stone of balance, strength and positive transformation. I love using it when I want to activate creativity and inspiration. It is an incredible balancing stone, as it evokes compassion and tolerance, while repelling and protecting from negative energy.

"Tiger's eye is the ultimate good luck charm. It works to power up your purpose with confidence and self-esteem. Like its namesake, it is the stone of strength, courage and inner strength.

"This trio of crystals works together, with the grounding power of connecting you with Mother Earth and to your energetic source, while helping you connect and work with your own intuitive, creative energy.

"Together, they help bring the boost of confidence to know you have what you need inside you to take your big, bold steps forward.

"You can place them in various places in and around the home or where you work. Be guided to where you intuitively feel you need those crystals and their energy to do their work. For example, placing them where you might work for a power up, or by the front door as an activator when you leave, or arrive home."

STEP SIX

HONOUR YOUR SELF-CARE

"There is a vitality, a life force, an energy, a quickening that is
translated through you into action, and because there is only one
of you in all of time, this expression is unique. And if you block it,
it will never exist through any other medium and it will be lost.
The world will not have it."

MARTHA GRAHAM

So far we've explored a whole world of coaching exercises, tools and strategies to help you feel empowered and in alignment for getting this BIG, BOLD, BEAUTIFUL show on the road, but if you aren't looking out for your wellbeing through self-care, things are going to be an uphill struggle from the get-go. Without wellbeing there's no energy for putting the BIG visions into being – who can set the world alight when all they want to do is have a nap?

The word "vitality" lands in a special place in my heart when it comes to this journey. It is the beating embodiment of what it is to live a BIG, BOLD, BEAUTIFUL life. The word itself stems from the latin word *vitalitas*, which translates to "vital force" or "life", "vitalis" meaning "belonging to life" and *vivere* "to live". To feel full of vitality to thrive within your BIG, BOLD, BEAUTIFUL existence.

Without vitality and wellbeing, there's no motivation or confidence for taking a BIG, BOLD, BEAUTIFUL stand for what you believe in, and leading a passionate cause for a better world. Without wellbeing you won't notice the wonder of the life you are crafting.

I'm mindful here that what wellbeing means for you, will look very different from what wellbeing looks like for me, or for anyone else in your world. Your wellbeing, and your approach to wellbeing and self-care, is as individual as you are. So, when it comes to creating a foundation of wellbeing in your BIG, BOLD, BEAUTIFUL life, you will find plenty of inspiration here that you can dive off from to find what works for you.

The approach to wellbeing in this step is all about compassionate self-care – being kind to yourself and devoting yourself to the level of individual care to honour the whole of you, as the wonderful human you are.

Wellbeing and self-care aren't just pithy hashtags. They are not a "nice-to-haves". They are a radical act of showing up for all of you. They are the vital force in your BIG, BOLD, BEAUTIFUL life, and will keep the fuel burning to help you create and live it.

Fold the corner of this page, or get a sticky marker and mark this step as one to come back to time and time again. Because this is where you put the *vitalitas* in the quest for your BIG, BOLD, BEAUTIFUL life.

IN STEP SIX YOU WILL:

✓ Discover the *eight pillars of self-care* and how they all interplay to help you live a BIG, BOLD, BEAUTIFUL life, and support you as you take action toward your vision with your soul goals.

✓ *Recognize your burnout symptoms* and signals. Explore some simple burnout remedies, which you can action straight away.

✓ Learn how to start thinking "self-care first" to *create moments of calm* (even among the chaos) for an empowered BIG, BOLD, BEAUTIFUL life.

✓ Find out about how to protect your energy and *activate your disco ball shine* to make sure you feel full of the right kind of energy to support your BIG, BOLD, BEAUTIFUL soul goals and journey.

✓ Celebrate the *power of rest* to fire up your potency, so that you can put more energy into what you are creating as you take action, and create space when you need it.

✓ Create a *self-care pledge* that will support you on every step of your BIG, BOLD, BEAUTIFUL journey and serve as a reminder of your wellbeing as a foundation to all that is your BIG, BOLD BEAUTIFUL life.

Ready to feel good and be well? Let's get to it!

THE EIGHT PILLARS OF SELF-CARE

In the same way you went on a 360 ride around your BIG, BOLD, BEAUTIFUL vision map, you can also go on a journey on a Wheel of Vitality as you experience eight key priority areas of wellbeing and self-care. In the Wheel of Vitality, the eight key priority areas are: mental, emotional, physical, spiritual, creative, recreational, social and environmental. Each interacts with the others to positively impact your overall wellbeing.

Let's explore each segment of the Wheel of Vitality.

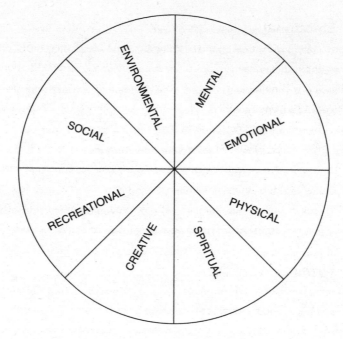

1. Mental (or psychological)

To be supported on this level is to create a healthy and cared for mind. This means creating awareness of the pressures that can cause overwhelm and burnout and addressing how you deal with adversity. Ultimately, your mental wellbeing is about finding ways to build a healthy mindset and some resilience techniques.

In the fast-paced, always-on world we live in, awareness of mental and psychological wellness is fundamental. I'm sure that you've found yourself stuck in over-thinking mode to the point where nothing seems clear. It's at these times when you're unable to take on anything else before it feels like you are going to fall down or fall over. Managing the mental load means freeing up some head space to be able to focus on your BIG, BOLD, BEAUTIFUL soul goals.

2. Emotional

From dealing with stresses and challenging situations, to life's ebbs and flows, through to healing from traumatic experiences, your emotional wellbeing means looking out for your emotional needs in any given moment, and any situation. Emotional wellbeing means honouring self-compassion, and fostering healthy boundaries, to support you in your BIG, BOLD, BEAUTIFUL life (as you uncovered in STEP FIVE).

There will have been times in your life when you have found it easier to cope. No doubt there have been other times when you've felt the world being pulled out from underneath you. Emotional wellbeing helps you find strategies for both ends of your emotional spectrum.

3. Physical

This involves how you take care of your physical vessel – from how much sleep you get, and the quality of that sleep, to how you nourish your body with nutrition and hydration, and what exercise supports your physical being, all the way through to prioritizing your gut health (p. 116). Your body is the physical manifestation of your life. To be supported in your BIG, BOLD, BEAUTIFUL life, you need your vessel to be looked after.

4. Spiritual

Being in alignment with your intuition, inner wisdom and connection to a deeper meaning for life, and how you live it, is vital. Spiritual wellbeing is connection to and curiosity about, that "something more" that's above and beyond your everyday reality, to help you tap in to a higher or deeper guidance.

Your spirituality can come from your beliefs, your faith or your values. It's where you find meaning in your BIG, BOLD, BEAUTIFUL life and life events – the golden breadcrumbs that make life make sense.

I like to think of spirituality as the inner dial that keeps your compass pointing in a direction of purpose and direction that feels true for you.

5. Creative

The essence of creativity is an essential flow of life. This isn't just about the act of creativity; it's the very essence of who you are, your creative self-expression, imagination and how you show up for your BIG, BOLD, BEAUTIFUL life. When you are dealing with stress and burnout, life can feel very uninspiring, and can trick you into thinking you've lost your spark.

Creativity is an essential element of your self-care. It reminds you of your purpose and powers up your resilience. It helps you tap into the limitless potential of life and provides you with endless ways to explore how you do things. It helps you to shift perspectives so you can find new ways to navigate the epic adventures and plot twists of your BIG, BOLD BEAUTIFUL journey.

6. Social

This is about having your joy squad ... your soul crew (p. 187). Building and nurturing meaningful and supportive relationships gives you the opportunity for your disco ball heart to shine. Your social self-care and wellbeing provides your sense of belonging and connection. It also brings the opportunity for growth, through diversity, respect, empathy, and encouragement of different perspectives and cultures.

7. Recreational

Without some downtime you are going to be one bored, exhausted human – no-one needs that! You can always work harder, and do more. You can always add more to your to-do list so that it becomes never-ending. Without having some time away from what you are focusing on, it can soon tip into overwhelm – so much so that all the enjoyment drains out of whatever you're doing.

Recreational downtime gives you breathing space, rest, reflection, inspiration, joy and play that will add more of the BIG, BOLD and BEAUTIFUL into your vision and goals.

8. Environmental

This is one that is so often over-looked, and yet the places and spaces you spend your time in, whether physical or energetic, have an incredible impact and influence on your wellbeing.

In the same way you wouldn't be able to do a workout on a factory floor, you will struggle to work on your BIG, BOLD, BEAUTIFUL soul goals if you are not in stimulating and supportive environments, near people who will help your BIG, BOLD, BEAUTIFUL life to flourish. It's why a lot of artists hire studio space so that they can work around other creatives.

So, now that you've taken a spin around the eight pillars of self-care on the Wheel of Vitality, find out how it gets to support you on the ride of your BIG, BOLD, BEAUTIFUL life.

EXERCISE

CREATE YOUR WHEEL OF VITALITY

You can use the same wheel format you used in STEP ONE (for your BIG, BOLD, BEAUTIFUL vision) to create your own Wheel of Vitality.

Use the wheel to check in on where you are in each area right now. The further away from the centre you position yourself, the better you feel you're doing in that area. It's likely that you might score low in some, if not most, areas to start with. Be curious. Notice where you score the lowest; that's what needs your more urgent attention.

Example:

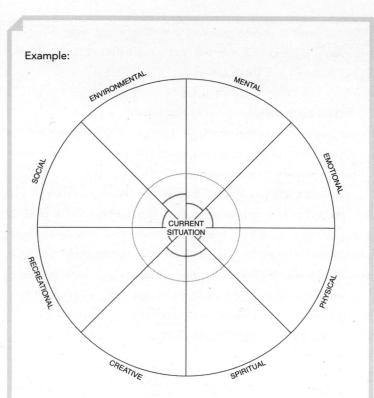

Then, come up with three simple actions in each area that could support your BIG, BOLD, BEAUTIFUL soul goals. In this example I would prioritize my goals for physical wellbeing because I score lowest in that segment of the wheel.

Example:

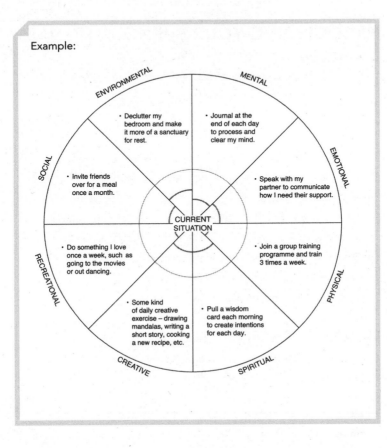

Your Wheel of Vitality is going to become your best friend as you explore what's next … which is where you might be in burning out.

RECOGNIZING YOUR BURNOUT SIGNALS

"She believed she could, but she was really tired,
so she didn't."
ANONYMOUS

One of the surest ways to pour water on the fire of your BIG, BOLD, BEAUTIFUL life is by being so exhausted and depleted that you can't seem to get anything going. I'm sure you've heard the often-hackneyed phrase, "You can't pour from an empty cup." It's used so much because it's so bloody true. But what happens when that cup has been empty for so long, you feel like you can barely set foot out of bed each day, let alone create a BIG, BOLD, BEAUTIFUL life?

It could be that you are in burnout.

WHAT IS BURNOUT?

Burnout is real. It is the manifestation of emotional, physical and mental exhaustion caused by prolonged exposure to stress. It's all the glaring warning signs, which show you that your mind, body and soul are waving a white flag, no longer able to cope with what's being thrown at you.

In 2019 the World Health Organization (WHO) included burnout in the 11th Revision of the International Classification of Diseases. They defined it as, "an occupational phenomenon resulting from chronic workplace stress that has not been successfully managed."

In an overwhelming always-on life, with pressures seeming to build year on year, burnout isn't just an occupational phenomenon that only affects workers in the workplace. It is reaching epidemic levels, in most places.

Burnout is the debilitating result of trying to carry too much, do too much, be all the things to all the people and make sure everyone else is OK ... while treading water in an over-stimulated, stress-filled, fear-fuelled world.

You may think you've been feeling more exhausted than normal. You might put it down to increased pressures of the world around you, and no matter what you do, that exhaustion isn't lifting. So, you learn to live with the symptoms – and adapt – rather than deal with what's going on underneath. If it feels like surviving, rather than thriving, it could be that you're already in burnout.

Common burnout symptoms:

- Fatigue and exhaustion of mind, body and soul
- Feeling tired and drained most of the time
- Inability to focus or concentrate
- Feeling disconnected and detached from the world
- Doubting yourself and your abilities
- Feeling hopeless or more cynical about the world
- Procrastinating, or things seem to take longer to do
- A lack of joy or sense of purpose
- Insomnia or disrupted sleep patterns
- Increased anxiety and even depression
- Feeling overwhelmed and unable to cope with even the simplest of tasks
- Crying more often / quicker to anger

Less common burnout symptoms:

- Feeling tired but over-stimulated (tired but wired)
- Compassion fatigue / apathy (no longer being able to give as much energy and empathy to those around you)
- Brain fog
- Getting more forgetful

- An increasing number of accidents
- Making more mistakes / doing seemingly stupid things like putting your car keys in the cutlery drawer and wondering why you can't find them!
- Seeming to get every cough, cold and virus going, because of a weakened immune system

How many of these symptoms do you connect with right now? They're not exactly the conditions conducive to living a BIG, BOLD, BEAUTIFUL life!

Burnout is not something that goes away on its own or with a week's holiday in the sunshine. It can have a real and debilitating impact on your life, so it's vital that you gain awareness of not just the symptoms of burnout that you might be experiencing, but what's causing the burnout.

And this may well be why you have sought out how to live a BIG, BOLD, BEAUTIFUL life in the first place. So, let's support that by getting underneath what could stop you – or hold you back – from doing so.

If you are in full burnout, deal with the burnout first, before you try and do anything toward your BIG, BOLD, BEAUTIFUL soul goals, so that:

1. You can start to get your health and your energy back (most importantly), and
2. You have enough energy to achieve your BIG, BOLD, BEAUTIFUL soul goals and to ensure you don't give up on your BIG, BOLD, BEAUTIFUL dreams because you're on your knees.

In this whole step of honouring your self-care you will find ways to support your wellbeing, which will help you if you're experiencing burnout.

Over the page you will find some simple burnout remedies and routines for immediate self-care.

BURNOUT REMEDIES FOR URGENT SELF-CARE

Seek support. There's no shame in admitting that you are struggling to cope. If you need to get help then you absolutely should. This might mean speaking to your doctor, a supportive work colleague or manager, a mental health first aider, or someone in your community who will be able to help you find the support you might need.

Down tools. If you find that you are experiencing burnout to the point that it's about to cross over into severe burnout then you have to stop. The likelihood that you are not doing things with full effectiveness, just blindly pushing on, is high … and it's a false economy.

Take time off. If you are working and experiencing burnout then you may need to take some time away from work. Speak to your manager, HR, or a health professional to discuss how you are feeling. Do it sooner rather than when it becomes too much to deal with.

Talk it out and get a plan. You may find talking therapies helpful to work through the pressures that are causing overwhelm in your life. A coach or therapist could help you find a plan to find strategies to get more ease in your life.

Get those endorphins pumping. Studies have found that aerobic exercise, such as running, weight training or cardio workouts, can help your brain recover from mental overwhelm and burnout.

Have fun! As hard as it might feel to find joy during burnout, doing things that bring you joy act as the leveller from the chronic stress you've been dealing with.

Depending on the level of your burnout your road to recovery may take longer than you initially expect it to. Remember, what's got you here could be years of build-up. The most important thing is to take it easy and do bite-sized things to recover. Keep checking in with how you're feeling.

CREATING MICRO-MOMENTS OF CALM AMONG THE CHAOS

The challenge is that we live in a world where self-care, and focusing on our wellbeing over productivity, has been viewed as an indulgence – guilty pleasures made up of long lunches, weekends away, day trips to a spa, or even the act of a long soak in the bath. It's time to change that narrative.

Self-care is not self-indulgent. It's not something you get around to when you have time, or for a special treat, or reward. Self-care is a fundamental part of your wellbeing. As such, when it comes to living a BIG, BOLD, BEAUTIFUL life, it has to be woven into the everyday fabric of your life.

Self-care can be as powerful as sitting with a cup of tea for five minutes of pure presence, which can often be more effective than meditating for an hour if you're likely to spend that hour getting distracted by what's on your to-do list.

If you find that you are putting off self-care, or leaving it until you have more time, or you feel more overwhelmed and busy than you've ever been, then this is the call of the disco ball to stop. Get off the crazy train … and breathe with me.

Just breathe.
Right here.
Right now.
Count down from five to one.
Slowly inhale on five, exhale on four, inhale on three, exhale on two, inhale on one.
Release with a soft and slow sigh.

You are not designed to operate at full speed, full tilt, all the time. This BIG, BOLD, BEAUTIFUL adventure is a journey for life, not a sprint to the finish line!

You can begin with self-care micro-moments, which can be as simple as doing things to meet your essential needs: keeping hydrated, eating well, getting a good sleep routine, taking a five minute break in between one task and the next – even building up to the old disco nap (a 20-minute power nap in the day).

Micro-moments are small interventions that you can put in place throughout the day, which can have a significant impact on your wellbeing – and ultimately on your productivity – by regulating your central nervous system. These moments of calm activate your parasympathetic nervous system, reducing your adrenaline and cortisol levels, along with your heart rate.

So, let's head on over and take a look at some ways you can bring micro-moments of self-care and wellbeing into your everyday routine, so you can be better equipped to get the energy in place that you need, to achieve your BIG, BOLD, BEAUTIFUL soul goals.

MICRO-MOMENTS OF CALM: FIVE-MINUTE WONDERS

Here's a starter list of suggestions for micro-moments of calm you can start bringing into practice right away:

Five-minute breath work: You can do these simple self-care breathing techniques while making a cup of tea or coffee, or even folding the washing.

- Square (or box) breath – Inhale for a count of four, hold for four, exhale for four, hold for four.
- 8, 4, 7 breathing – Inhale deeply (and loudly) through your mouth for a count of eight, carry on inhaling through your nose for four, exhale for seven.
- Five-finger breathing exercise – Hold one hand in front of you with your fingers spread. Trace the outside of your hand with the index finger of your other hand. Breathe as you trace your finger up, then exhale as you trace down.

Five-minute technology break: Down tools and do something else. Scrolling does not count as a break!

Five-minute work break: Take a five-minute break before each task or meeting, or a five-minute break afterwards. Schedule in that time to make sure you get some space between one thing and the next.

Outside for five: Take your shoes off and connect to the earth. Feel connected and grounded.

Listen for five: Put your headphones on and listen to a soothing piece of music.

Dance for five: Put your headphones on or turn your speakers up and have a good old boogie.

Shake for five: Put some lively music on, and shake your body for five minutes! (This has so many health and emotional benefits.)

Body scan for five: Sit in a chair or lie down and breathe awareness into each part of your body. Start with your toes on one foot and then work your way up one side of your body, then down the other, name each part of your body in your mind as you do so.

Mindful for five … four … three … two … one: Practise this simple mindfulness technique (it's one of my favourites). Start by noticing five things you can hear, see, touch or feel, smell and even taste (this is great with something like a piece of chocolate or fruit). Then, think of four things you can hear, see, feel, smell and taste, then three, then two, then one.

Over to you! I've shared a whole lot of inspiration. What micro-moment ideas can you come up with to bring into your day?

My five-minute micro-moments of calm:

....

....

....

....

....

Now that you've explored your micro-moments of calm, it's time to work on your energetic wellbeing …

MAKING YOUR DISCO BALL SHINE

As you discovered with your self-empowerment toolkit, when it comes to exploring your boundaries, there are going to be people, places and spaces that fill you up and those that drain you. When it comes to mastering self-care, having an awareness of how you protect and perceive your own energy – by practising good energy hygiene – is going to help you feel well and be well in places and spaces that support you.

And OK, it's not always as easy as removing yourself from people and places that seem to take everything out of you – those pesky energy vampires! But you can practise protecting your energy before you have to be around those people – and in those environments – that drain you. Your disco ball shine is your glorious heart and the BIG, BOLD, BEAUTIFUL energy you exude to the world. It's time to polish it up and keep that disco ball full of light and sparkle!

EXERCISE

DRAIN OR BOOST?

First off is to gain awareness of where you feel your energy gets drained, and where it gets boosted, and then explore energy protection, clearing and boosting techniques. That's what you will find in the energy protection exercises in the next section.

Explore your energy drains and boosts:

WHAT DRAINS ME:

People:

Example: A co-worker who never has anything positive to say.

....

....

Places:

Example: My work environment has a toxic blame culture.

....

....

Spaces:

Example: My home office is too dark, and looks out onto a brick wall.

....

....

WHAT LIFTS ME:

People:

Example: My best friend who's always got the best advice and makes me feel great.

....

....

Places:

Example: Ibiza! The colour of the landscapes, the people, the energy and the vibe. It's my happy place.

....

....

Spaces:

Example: My home, which is filled with people and things that I love, and happy memories I have collected through the years.

....

....

LIGHT UP YOUR DISCO BALL! IDEAS FOR ENERGY PROTECTION

Start with these simple ideas and techniques for protecting your energy around people, places and spaces. Then, come up with some ideas of your own that you can bring into your self-care routine:

CREATE A POWER WORD OR MANTRA

As you have already explored – words have power – so find an energetic power word that resonates deeply with you. This could be one word that always makes you feel super-charged or a mantra, which is a word or phrase that's chanted, usually as part of a meditation practice.

Power words can be related to your values, such as FREEDOM, ADVENTURE, JOY. Or they can be mantras in and of themselves, such as Om (Aum), the Sanskrit vibrational word that represents the creation of the Universe or Ram, the vibrational mantra that is linked to the solar plexus chakra to help you feel more empowered.

ZIP IT UP

Imagine zipping yourself up inside an energetic power bubble that has all of the things in it that keep you feeling full of vitality and confidence. Plus, it keeps out anything that doesn't.

TAKE A RAINBOW LIGHT SHOWER

Protective energy can come in the form of colour and light. This can be related to chakras, and their associated energy. Chakras are energetic centres within the physical and energetic body, which allow universal life force, or *Prana* (in Sanskrit) to flow in and around the body. Each chakra is related to physical, emotional and psychological wellbeing, which allows that vital life force energy to move through all aspects of our physiological and energetic flow.

The seven key chakras of the body help to activate BIG, BOLD, BEAUTIFUL energy to sustain and support you. These are:

- Root chakra – Red for grounding, stabilizing, protective
- Sacral – Orange for relationship to self, sensuality, unconscious creativity
- Solar plexus – Yellow/gold for inner power, confidence, purpose
- Heart – Green/pink for love, compassion, relationship with others
- Throat – Blue for communication, being heard, speaking truth
- Third Eye (brow) – Violet/purple for insight, intuition, self-trust
- Crown – Ultra-violet, white, silver for connection, spirituality, trust in the Universe

Now imagine taking all of that incredible energy and showering in it! You can literally do this anywhere – on public transport, in a supermarket queue. Here's how:

- Close your eyes. Breathe deeply.
- Imagine the colour red showering down on you and around you. It's creating a dome of colour, all the way around you and underneath you.
- Then the orange is showering down, creating the next layer of colour.
- Then yellow/gold, followed by green or pink, then blue, then violet and purple ... followed by the final colour of ultraviolet, white or silver, to seal you in with seven colours of rainbow energy that you can take with you everywhere.

CLEAR YOUR PHYSICAL AND ENERGETIC SPACE

Clear and declutter your space of the physical – mess, paperwork, clothes, etc., and energetic – objects that hold negative energy or emotions, such as old photos, journals and diaries, even down to people when they've been in your space!

You can cleanse your energy space, using smoke and smudge sticks, incense or dried plants such as juniper, rosemary and cedar. Make sure you have a door or a window open so that everything you are clearing has a place to leave through.

Fill your space with things that bring you joy as well as powerful and positive energy. Plants are great for this, as well as photos of joyful memories, art that you love, or motivating quotes and prints.

Now that your space and your energy is becoming clearer, you can dive deeper into your wellbeing journey by activating the power of rest.

THE SUPERPOWER OF REST

Rest is the elixir that gives your brain, body and energy the space to recuperate and replenish. It also gives your mind the chance to recharge and restore all that creative power energy as you take steps toward your BIG, BOLD, BEAUTIFUL soul goals.

The truth is that in the busy, overwhelming and often distracting world that we live in – with decisions to be made, things to do, plans to be fulfilled – it's very easy to hit mental and energetic congestion. Trying to squeeze anything else into this overwhelm factory, by doing more, ultimately makes you less productive.

Rest is the antidote to this.

- It is the literal breathing space that allows your ideas and BIG, BOLD, BEAUTIFUL soul goals to take shape.
- It activates the parasympathetic nervous system, to bring your body repair.
- It can help with building neural pathways in the brain, developing new skills and enhancing creativity and learning.
- It improves your overall mental and physical health by reducing blood pressure and boosting your immune system.

As short and sweet as this is … all in all, rest is your superpower of self-care, and an essential part of living and creating within your BIG, BOLD, BEAUTIFUL life.

Explore more below for some BIG, BOLD, BEAUTIFUL rest techniques.

POWERING UP YOUR REST
Take rest days

In the same way you would have rest days if you were on an exercise regime, taking rest days from your BIG, BOLD, BEAUTIFUL soul goals and anything you have on your plate right now, is fundamental.

Rest days mean doing anything other than working, or even the household chores. They are days where you can rest, be, explore, and spend time on leisure activities to top yourself back up.

What might your rest days activities look like?

Example: "A day out in nature walking the dog and exploring somewhere I haven't been before."

....

....

Fire up your love vibe levels

Oxytocin is the feel-good bonding hormone, otherwise known as the "cuddle hormone" or "love hormone". It has been found to lower stress and anxiety levels and regulate emotional responses, as well as helping to build trust, empathy, positive memories and communication. It's the ultimate wellbeing super-boost.

Ways to boost your oxytocin:

- Pet a dog. Research has shown that both dogs and humans see an increase in oxytocin from physical contact, including patting and stroking.
- Intimacy. This includes cuddling, hugging, kissing, holding hands.
- Touch. Self-massage, giving or receiving a massage from someone else.
- Making love. Self-pleasure and masturbation also fall under this heading.
- Dancing.
- Singing in a group.
- Listening to your favourite music.
- Watching a feel-good movie.
- Preparing a meal and sharing food. (Figs, watermelon, avocados, broccoli, chia seeds, dark chocolate and green tea all naturally boost oxytocin.)

Practise waking rest

Waking rest is a great mindful meditation practice. It gives space for calm, by allowing a conscious space to allow your mind to wander, meaning that it has a chance to filter the mundane everyday thoughts that take up so much brain space. Did you know that the brain takes up 20% of your overall energetic power battery each day?

Amanda Lamp of Washington State University describes waking rest as "... A period of quiet, reflective thought that allows the brain time to consider and process whatever arises spontaneously."

You can start with 2 – 3 minutes each morning before you leap out of bed. This should let the thoughts of your sleep, or what you have in front of you in your day, to filter. Build up to 5 – 15 minutes, which can be done while you are doing everyday tasks such as folding washing, cleaning your teeth, showering or walking the dog.

How to practise waking rest:

- Give yourself time to explore your thoughts while you're doing a low-energy mundane task. (Steer clear of doing this while watching television or scrolling on social media.)
- Let your thoughts take the lead. You could think about what you are doing in the day ahead, the dreams you've just had, reflect on old happy memories and past experiences, check in on where you are now, or daydream about the future.
- Let your thoughts come up. Don't force new ideas or directions.
- Don't judge what comes up, either. Just let thoughts percolate and wash through. (This is great if you take your waking rest in the shower as you can let them wash down the plughole!)

Take a digital detox

You knew it was coming ... The digital detox isn't just about putting your mobile onto airplane mode overnight; it's about having time away from all devices and screens. This will give your nervous system a chance to recalibrate, give your brain and your adrenals a break, and help to balance your emotional state and mood.

Simple ways to digitally detox:

- Schedule some time away from screens each day.
- Get out – go for a walk, or outside with a cuppa.
- Eat lunch away from your house / office. (Just make sure you don't take your phone with you!)

Other ways to digitally detox

Delete email and social media apps from your phone.
Email and social media are likely to be the biggest draws to your devices, so in your downtime (evenings and weekends) remove the apps that are most likely to make you want to hit the home screen.

Downgrade your phone.
There's an increasing demand for phones that you can only phone and text from. This is a great way to cut down on the amount of time you spend on a device in any given day.

Lock your work devices away overnight, or over the weekend.
If you have devices specifically for work, have a place where you can put your laptop or mobile away, so you have to consciously make an effort to get them out when you are on downtime from work.

Make use of your phone's features.
Depending on your make and model of phone you can take advantage of the do not disturb, focus or sleep functions to make sure you're not getting calls or notifications that will make you want to reach for them.

You can also use the phone's function that limits the amount of time you spend on particular apps.

Turn your devices off at a specific time each day.
You may choose to turn your devices off at dinner time in the evening, or an hour before you go to bed, to make sure you've had enough time away from screens.

Create a no-device area.
As long as the temptation is there you will always be tempted to reach for your devices. It could be useful to have your dedicated rest space free from all devices. Not only will it create better conditions for sleep, it will stop mindless scrolling, or checking that last-minute email before bed – or on waking up!

Now that you've explored all of the great tools and techniques to honour your self-care here in STEP SIX, my hope is that you will go on a deeper adventure into wellbeing and self-care, to discover more and find even more practices and techniques that work for you on your BIG, BOLD, BEAUTIFUL journey.

COMMITTING TO SELF-CARE

Your commitment to your BIG, BOLD, BEAUTIFUL LIFE is a commitment to honouring yourself and your wellbeing. Everything that is shared in these pages creates the ideal container for your success. That success depends on you and how you show up for yourself. Honouring yourself is the essential element to it all.

Committing to self-care and coming back to it often will be the wind beneath the wings of your BIG, BOLD, BEAUTIFUL journey – and your life. One of the best ways to do this is by creating a pledge of commitment to self-care as part of your BIG, BOLD, BEAUTIFUL life. Head on over to the next exercise to create your Self-care Pledge.

EXERCISE

CREATE A SELF-CARE PLEDGE

What follow are the prompts to help you create your Self-care Pledge, which follows the Wheel of Vitality you explored at the beginning of STEP SIX. The idea is to commit to making self-care a priority.

How you create your pledge is up to you. You can get as creative as you like. The more visual the better. I have mine as a big wall planner that I colour-code and stick inspiring images onto. The most important thing to do is to print it out, or create it in a way that means you can see it each and every day, so that you can check in and come back to it often.

This pledge is something that every person who comes onto the Kickstart Your BIG, BOLD, BEAUTIFUL Life Programme creates before they start exploring their BIG, BOLD, BEAUTIFUL vision.

Explore the prompts and get creative with your Self-care Pledge:

MY COMMITMENT TO MENTAL WELLBEING

Example: "Take regular mental health breaks. Make sure that I am not taking too much on. If I have too many tabs open in my brain I will find ways to take something off my plate and focus on one thing at a time."

....

....

....

MY COMMITMENT TO EMOTIONAL WELLBEING

Example: "Practise self-compassion on a regular basis, through daily gratitude, journalling, meditation and increasing my oxytocin levels. When I get into negative self-talk, I will speak kindly to myself and find ways to reframe whatever my inner critic is telling me."

....

....

....

MY COMMITMENT TO PHYSICAL WELLBEING

Example: "Move my body and boost my mind each day, with some form of exercise, even if it's just for 10 minutes. Try weight training for strength and stamina, yoga for core strength and flexibility, Qoya for a good dance, shake and my overall wellness."

....

....

....

MY COMMITMENT TO SPIRITUAL WELLBEING

Example: "Get out into nature each day to ground myself and connect. Spend time creating intentions by journalling each day. Seek out new experiences and classes to explore with a beginner's mindset. Find something new to explore, on a bi-monthly basis."

....

....

....

MY COMMITMENT TO CREATIVE WELLBEING

Example: "Explore writing poetry and reading for pleasure; this gives me so much inspiration. Listen to new music. Sign up to that pottery class!" (That's a note to self too!)

....

....

....

MY COMMITMENT TO RECREATIONAL WELLBEING

Example: "Take downtime to do things that feel like play, such as sea swimming, dancing or going to a gig. I can also explore new things this way."

....

....

....

MY COMMITMENT TO SOCIAL WELLBEING

Example: "Plan a monthly hangout with my closest friends so we can have lunch or dinner together, catch up and stay connected. Invite friends to join me at the events I book, based on what they also enjoy, as well as being open to meeting new like-minded people."

....

....

....

MY COMMITMENT TO ENVIRONMENTAL WELLBEING

Example: "Spend time each weekend honouring my home/bedroom/ office spaces by decluttering/cleaning and cleansing. I will spend at least one day per week working in a different environment."

....

....

....

Now that you've created your Self-care Pledge, come back to it often, and put the things you've pledged into action!

STEP SIX REVIEW TIME

So, here we are at the close of STEP SIX, honouring your self-care and wellbeing to put the vitality into your BIG, BOLD, BEAUTIFUL life. Keep exploring and keep coming back to the self-care tools and techniques you've learned about here.

Here's a handy checklist of SELF-CARE tools and exercises you can come back to, to create a wellbeing plan that works alongside your BIG, BOLD, BEAUTIFUL soul goals, and when you need a wellbeing boost:

✓ Create your *Wheel of Vitality* to connect to the eight pillars of self-care, support your wellbeing, and give vital energy to your BIG, BOLD, BEAUTIFUL vision.

✓ Check in on any *burnout symptoms and signals* and put some some remedies into action for when you need a spot of urgent self-care.

✓ Create *micro-moments of calm*, with exercises that can lead to sustainable, everyday self-care routines.

✓ Let your *disco ball shine*, and get a BIG, BOLD, BEAUTIFUL energy boost with exercises that will keep you vibrating and shining bright.

✓ Tap into the *super-power of rest*.

And finally, and probably most importantly of all …

✓ Create your *Self-care Pledge*, so that you have an active reminder of what will help you to feel full of vitality and vibrancy every step of the way, as you take action on your soul goals and take each step toward your BIG, BOLD, BEAUTIFUL vision and life.

And so, onto the very last step on this BIG, BOLD, BEAUTIFUL journey – STEP SEVEN, where we will explore the magical power of celebration before popping the champagne corks on our time together and getting the glitter cannons primed for the next part of your BIG, BOLD, BEAUTIFUL adventure.

Before you dive in, head on over to the BIG, BOLD, BEAUTIFUL Breakout Ritual, to explore some blissful five-minute meditations.

BREAKOUT RITUAL
FIVE-MINUTE MEDITATIONS

Meditation doesn't have to mean getting up an hour earlier each day or clearing space in your diary to make it happen. It also doesn't mean completely clearing your mind. Creating space in your everyday, by creating a ritual, can be a meditation practice in and of itself. It can be as simple as taking five minutes out to honour your intuition and pause for breath.

Below are some beautiful meditation and ritual practices that you can weave into each and every day, to honour your self-care, and also give you a moment to reflect on what you are achieving and honouring as you move through your BIG, BOLD, BEAUTIFUL soul goals.

While most meditations require you to close your eyes and focus your attention inwards, these meditations are different. They're based on *Trataka*, which means "to look", or "gaze", in Sanskrit. The idea is that through the act of gazing, you activate the pineal gland, associated with opening up your inner wisdom and intuition.

CANDLE GAZING MEDITATION

- Find yourself some space where you will be undisturbed. This one works best if you're in a dimly lit or darkened room.
- Light a candle.
- Sit somewhere where you can be at eye level with the candle, making sure you are comfortable.
- Focus your attention and gaze on the flame.
- Hold your gaze there. If you find your eyes or your mind wandering then bring your attention back to the flame.
- Try to keep your eyes open. Your eyes may water, but this will pass. If you do blink bring your attention back to the flame.
- Keep breathing deeply and focus on the light with each inhale and exhale.
- Keep going until your only awareness is of the flame.
- When this is complete, blow out the candle and either lie down, or stay seated. Close your eyes for a few minutes and then allow your mind and body to come back to awareness before you continue with your day.

BUDDHIST WATER GAZING MEDITATION

- This is similar to the candle gazing meditation, but it's one you can do when you are out in nature near a body of water, such as a river or a lake. It works well if the water is gently flowing or still rather than choppy.
- Find yourself somewhere peaceful to sit where you will not be disturbed.
- Get into a comfortable position, where you can sit connected to the earth.
- Gaze into the water and breathe deeply.
- Notice the shape, flow and movement of the water.
- Notice the light reflecting from the water.
- Notice how it ebbs and flows.

- Try to keep your gaze fixed on the water. If your eyes wander, or you blink, bring your attention back to a spot on the water.
- Focus on the gentle movement or stillness of the light and the water with each breath.
- Keep gazing into the water, until you feel you are in complete connection and flow with it.
- When you feel your meditation is complete, you can close your eyes for a few minutes to bring your mind and body back to awareness, before moving on.

CLOUD OR SKY GAZING

This is one of the most simple and pleasurable gazing meditations you can enjoy. Sky gazing is a key practice from the Dzogchen tradition of Tibetan Buddhism. It emphasizes the idea that we already have everything we need within us. Being connected to the sky, and the clouds, reminds us to connect with something greater than us, and the infinite potential of the sky.

You can carry out the practice of sky or cloud gazing in your garden, when you are outdoors, through a window, or as a passenger in a car or a train. (It's even better when you are in an aeroplane that's sitting above the clouds.) Basically, you can do it anywhere you can get a good view of the sky and the clouds.

As before, make sure you are comfortable and your back is supported, or that you have something to lie down on if you prefer.

If you are around other people you may want to have some headphones on, either playing some soft music, or simply blocking out the noise around you.

- Breathe deeply and look up to the clouds in the sky.
- Take notice of the shapes they form, how they move, how they change.
- Don't get too hung up on trying to make out any specific shapes; just notice what you notice.

- Notice how fast, slowly or gently they move, and what direction they are moving in.
- Notice how effortlessly they move and change shape.
- Take notice of how each cloud is unique.
- As they change shape or dissolve let your thoughts and feelings dissolve with them and with every breath you exhale.
- If any thoughts or tensions arise, send them off into the clouds, to disperse and change form.
- Take notice of any new ideas that might come to you.
- When you feel your meditation is complete, you can close your eyes for a few minutes to bring your mind and body back to awareness, before finishing this practice and journalling on any new ideas that came up for you during it.

Just a note: if you are outdoors for either the water gazing or cloud gazing meditations, make sure you are wearing adequate eye and skin sun protection, even on a cloudy day.

STEP SEVEN

HARNESS THE POWER OF SELF-CELEBRATION

Here we are, you glorious disco ball hearted human, on the final step as you high-kick it into your BIG, BOLD, BEAUTIFUL life. What a ride … and it's not over yet! In this final fling on the BIG, BOLD, BEAUTIFUL epic, you are going to explore how to harness the power of celebration and its essential role in creating and living your BIG, BOLD, BEAUTIFUL life. We do this, not just because I love a glitter cannon (this much is true), but because celebration has a crucial role to play in staying the course on this BIG, BOLD, BEAUTIFUL path.

Without celebration there's just hustle and hard work.

As you dance your way to BIGGER, BOLDER and even more BEAUTIFUL opportunities, you grow, shift and expand, and with them celebration becomes the energy, motivation, momentum and inspiration behind all the incredible work you are doing.

At the pinnacle of this guide to living a BIG, BOLD, BEAUTIFUL life you are going to learn how celebration interplays with gratitude and positive psychology. You will celebrate every step of your journey as well as seeking out everyday ways to bring celebration into your BIG, BOLD, BEAUTIFUL way of being.

IN STEP SEVEN YOU WILL:

✓ Discover why *celebrating is for life, not just birthdays or special occasions,* and how it holds up a mirror to your strength, resilience and magic that becomes a life force as you move through your BIG, BOLD, BEAUTIFUL soul goals and journey.

✓ Explore why *celebration is good for your health* and wellbeing – and how adding celebration as part of taking action on your soul goals, and within every aspect of your BIG, BOLD, BEAUTIFUL life, is a radical way of practising empowering loving self-care.

✓ Don your pom-poms to *become your own cheerleader,* through the power of self-celebration, to build confidence, self-acceptance, positive energy and a vibrational shift in alignment with your BIG, BOLD, BEAUTIFUL goals and vision.

✓ Get on down with *everyday celebration,* to discover simple and effective ways to celebrate the small wins, each time you take action on your soul goals and with every step toward your BIG, BOLD, BEAUTIFUL LIFE.

✓ Learn about the powerful energetic frequency of gratitude so you can *activate your disco ball heart* as the ultimate act of love for your BIG, BOLD, BEAUTIFUL life. Find out how a simple daily gratitude practice can bring your BIG, BOLD, BEAUTIFUL vision into embodied being.

Let's fire up the confetti cannons, and explore this final step with all the sparkle and vibes, bringing this BIG, BOLD, BEAUTIFUL party to a close with a glitter-filled bang.

CELEBRATING IS FOR LIFE, NOT JUST FOR SPECIAL OCCASIONS

"The more you praise and celebrate your life,
the more there is in life to celebrate."
OPRAH WINFREY

Imagine taking every step you've taken on your BIG, BOLD, BEAUTIFUL life – every milestone reached, every hurdle or obstacle you've overcome, every challenge you've faced – and not acknowledging how far you've come or what you've achieved. Imagine ignoring every miracle and magical thing that comes your way, or looking past every experience you're having on this BIG, BOLD, BEAUTIFUL journey. How much impact do you think this would have on your ability to keep going, to know how far you've come, to set yourself up for the rest of the journey? It's going to get pretty tough to keep going, right? You're likely to wonder if it's possible for you to get what it is you so desire in your BIG, BOLD, BEAUTIFUL life, or question if it's even worth doing.

My guess is that you're reading this wondering if you *ever* take the time to notice or appreciate all of the parts you've had to play in getting you to where you are now. Or, whether you've noticed that every time something incredible has happened in your life, you had a fundamental role in making that happen. Or, how every failure you've had in your life, you've learned from.

And I'm going out on a limb to say that you might look at the things you've done and achieved and tell yourself stories about how you could have done things better; how you should have done more; how you feel like however much you do it's not enough – you are not enough. Speaking from one over-achiever, to another – I see you.

When any of these scenarios are happening we are training the brain and unconscious mind that what we do doesn't really matter because no matter what you do, nothing is ever really good enough.

Not exactly BIG, BOLD or BEAUTIFUL, right?

I'm calling it out, not so you can be even harder on yourself, but to highlight what happens when you are not celebrating yourself and your achievements. Celebration is a recognition of how far you've come and all the incredible resolve, determination, strength, resilience and power you have within you.

It brings out the best in you.

It will show you just how capable you really are.

How you've always been enough …

… More than enough.

Celebration will give you the energy, spirit, drive and determination that will help you with every step toward your BIG, BOLD, BEAUTIFUL vision. It is the extra tool to have in place to keep you from chasing every shiny squirrel that comes your way, and will keep you feeling optimistic and excited about your BIG, BOLD, BEAUTIFUL vision.

It helps you create BIGGER.

It puts the BOLD into your being.

It helps you to recognize how BEAUTIFUL the life you are creating is.

There's so much to love about pulling the proverbial party poppers on your BIG, BOLD, BEAUTIFUL adventures, and I consider it to be one of the most essential ingredients of a BIG, BOLD, BEAUTIFUL life, rather than merely an afterthought. In the next section, delve deeper to uncover the power of self-celebration and its wellbeing benefits.

CELEBRATING IS GOOD FOR YOUR HEALTH
(AND BIG, BOLD, BEAUTIFUL ENERGY)

Anyone who knows me knows I will find any excuse to throw confetti around, and with good reason. Once you understand the benefits of celebrating, you will wonder why you haven't been doing it before! In fact celebrating is so good for us that studies have shown that celebrating and practising gratitude have a profoundly positive impact on our physical, mental and emotional health. Here are just some of the benefits:

Physical

- Boosts your immune system
- Lowers blood pressure and increases heart health
- Improves your quality of sleep
- Counterbalances symptoms of burnout

Mental

- Counters negative emotions and reprogrammes toward increased levels of positive emotions
- Increases the production of serotonin and dopamine, the feel-good and reward hormones
- Reduces stress by lowering cortisol and adrenaline levels
- Has been found to reduce symptoms of depression and anxiety

Emotional

- Boosts confidence, self-acceptance and resilience
- Increases feelings of joy and pleasure, optimism and overall happiness
- Increases life satisfaction and feelings of contentment, fulfillment and peace
- Helps you to feel more outgoing and connected to others

I have witnessed time and again the magical flick of the switch when my clients start focusing on all of the incredible things that are happening as they hot-step it through their BIG, BOLD, BEAUTIFUL life. They literally light up – their eyes sparkle, their shoulders drop and they stand taller in the knowledge that they can, and they are, putting the BIG, the BOLD and the BEAUTIFUL into their lives. Once this awareness is seen, felt and reflected, they literally start banking the energy and power that celebration brings them, ready to call upon it when they need it on the BIG, BOLD, BEAUTIFUL journey ahead.

Of course, celebration has to come from the willingness to accept that you are worthy of celebrating your achievements, and being open to receiving the positive benefits celebration is going to bring into your life. This can often be one of the hardest things to do; it's all too easy to put our achievements down to luck, divine timing, or even pass it off as someone else's success.

Celebrating is a radical act of self-love and acceptance.

In the next exercise you are going to learn a gentle practice of loving self-acceptance through celebration.

EXERCISE

LOVING SELF-ACCEPTANCE THROUGH CELEBRATION

This is an opportunity to get curious and celebrate your strengths and "weaknesses",* which so often prove to be two sides of the same coin. Through this exercise you will gain a more holistic perspective of what you will bring to your BIG, BOLD, BEAUTIFUL journey, and how you can ultimately celebrate all of yourself and who you are in your BIG, BOLD, BEAUTIFUL life.

*I will always use inverted commas because every "weakness" is a negative self-imposed view of ourselves.

The idea is that – through this practice – you will discover more about all parts of yourself from a place of wholeness and self-acceptance.

CELEBRATE YOUR STRENGTHS

YOUR STRENGTHS	HOW THEY SUPPORT YOU	SELF-ACCEPTANCE CELEBRATION TIME
Example: I am great at coming up with new ideas.	I am a creative thinker.	I celebrate my creativity. The fact that I am a creative thinker, means I can always find a new solution and opportunities in any challenge.

Now, observe the other side, for a different perspective and how you can celebrate this too.

CELEBRATE YOUR "WEAKNESSES"

YOUR "WEAKNESSES"	LEARNINGS ABOUT THEM / ACTIONS YOU CAN TAKE	SELF-ACCEPTANCE CELEBRATION TIME
Example: I sometimes have so many ideas that I struggle to get one thing finished. I can get distracted easily. Ultimately, this hinders my progress toward my BBB vision. I'm all ideas and little action!	I need to be creatively stimulated, and things need to feel new and exciting, but in alignment with my original BBB vision. I can get support for the things that I find boring.	I am a creative thinker, which is a strength. I can play to my strengths to keep things feeling creative and exciting and get help for the things that don't hold my attention.

Keeping returning to this exercise as you delve deeper on the BIG, BOLD, BEAUTIFUL journey. It's incredibly powerful for you to witness that you have strengths where you didn't know they existed, and that even your "weaknesses" have a powerful energy to them. For now, let's take this warm up in the celebration gym, and dive deeper into the power of self-celebration for your BIG, BOLD, BEAUTIFUL adventures ahead.

BECOMING YOUR BIGGEST CHAMPION

It's time to pick up your pom-poms and create your own celebration cheer, as we get down with the power of self-celebration. You'll build confidence and self-acceptance, and provide bundles of positive energy as you disco dance your way toward your BIG, BOLD, BEAUTIFUL life, by taking stock of everything you are doing to make it happen.

Self-celebration is a way of acknowledging the part you play in what you are creating, reinforcing your achievements, rather than pushing them away or pushing on through. As the wonderful Sarah Powell, Founder of Celebrate Yourself, describes self celebration as, "Discovering, choosing and having the best relationship you can with yourself. It is finding ways to tap in to your self-compassion, show yourself kindness, know your self-worth and be able to support, honour, accept and like, even love, yourself."

Self-celebration is another powerful tool to have in your self-empowerment toolkit as you navigate your BIG, BOLD, BEAUTIFUL journey. It can lead to healthier and better conversations with your inner critic when it pipes up to tell you all the things you're failing at, which it will ... *I bet you can drag up something shitty that happened over 10 years ago, quicker than you can draw on three brilliant things that happened on the same day!*

But it's not all about celebrating the big wins or milestones, as Sarah goes on to say, "You don't need to be 'fixed' or change everything so that you can celebrate yourself. Instead, you can celebrate and honour the person you are right now, exactly as you are. It provides an alternative to your inner critic and fixating on shortcomings and failures, and instead focuses on supporting yourself. And it exists in the small day-to-day actions. The way we treat and speak to ourselves, THAT is self-celebration. It's quiet and super powerful."

So you see, when you celebrate yourself and your actions and achievements, you reinforce the behaviour you want to show up when you are doing something new ... so much so that you can anchor the positive behaviour into the body.

So, now that you've discovered why celebrating is for all of your BIG, BOLD, BEAUTIFUL life, let's discover how you can bring celebration into the every day of it.

EVERY DAY IS CAUSE FOR CELEBRATION

One of the things that stops most people celebrating their actions, and the steps they've taken toward their BIG, BOLD, BEAUTIFUL life, is that they just don't know *how* to celebrate. This can be because there's an association that celebration is wild and extravagant, or that it needs to cost time and money. More than that, many people have a sense that celebration is "allowed" only once the work is all done. But truth is, that often the work is never complete, it simply evolves into something else. So, unless what you're woking on has a very defined measure of "success" and completion, then celebration can never happen.

Your BIG, BOLD, BEAUTIFUL life is one that's always evolving. Your vision and soul goals will change. They will shift, grow and develop as you do, so unless you are taking notice of all of the things that are getting you where you are going, you will feel like you are on a constant treadmill of hustle. Instead, what we are exploring through celebration is the recognition of the incredible amount of energy and power in the small wins, actions and achievements.

When you celebrate the small wins as part of an everyday practice, not only are you getting all those juicy dopamine hits, your brain is lighting up synapses like an illumination parade! The more your brain is having its own celebratory party, the more it rewires to seek out more of the good stuff. Celebrating the small wins literally retrains your brain to seek out more achievement and rewards. Take that, negative bias!

Celebrating the small wins also feeds the brain and helps you take notice of the power of what you are putting in to make your BIG, BOLD, BEAUTIFUL vision come to life. As you create conscious awareness of your wins, you are creating a vibrational shift from lack, "Nothing ever works out for me. What's the point?" – to abundance and energetic elevation, "Anything is possible. If I can do this, imagine what else I can do." As you celebrate your wins, you are attracting more of what you are putting out on an energetic level. BIG, BOLD, BEAUTIFUL manifestation in action!

Celebrating the small wins is not all popping champagne corks and extravagant treats. It can be in the simple everyday actions of taking notice and marking them when they happen. What's even more important is to build them into your BIG, BOLD, BEAUTIFUL soul goals. So, ask yourself, "How will I celebrate?" as you are planning out your micro-actions. (Head on back to STEP TWO for a reminder of how to build these into the actions you are taking toward your soul goals.)

Go to the next page, for some simple ways to celebrate, each time you take action toward your BIG, BOLD, BEAUTIFUL life.

CELEBRATING THE SMALL WINS

One of the hardest things about the act of celebration is finding ways to actually celebrate. So I've gathered celebrations from those who've been Kickstart Your BIG, BOLD, BEAUTIFUL Life Programme, so you have some simple and effective ideas. Get ready to pay tribute to all those small wins and micro-actions you are taking that make up every step on the path to your BIG, BOLD, BEAUTIFUL life.

20 ideas for everyday celebration:

1. Create a celebration power playlist and have a celebratory dance.
2. Take a mindful break and explore what you've achieved.
3. Give yourself some downtime.
4. Get outside and connect with the celebration of nature – a big old flower in bloom, the sun in the sky, the trees full of leaves.
5. Have a nap (one of my personal faves).
6. Buy, or send yourself, some flowers.
7. Write yourself a celebration love note.
8. Take yourself out for lunch/celebratory cake!
9. Order in takeout or your favourite food.
10. Read a chapter of your book (preferably with a lovely cuppa and some of your favourite chocolate)!
11. Enjoy a glass of fizz (or your favourite tipple).
12. Write a list of things you love spending time doing. Pick something off that list for the sheer heck of enjoying it.
13. Hang out with your joy machine of a pet or favourite human!
14. Be spontaneous.
15. Celebrate with those who helped you make it possible.
16. Have a spa treatment. This could either mean taking time for an at-home treatment or going out to get something done.
17. Take a selfie – celebrate this moment in time, so you can go back to it and remind yourself how great it felt.
18. Take yourself out to the movies to watch a film you want to watch, or watch one of your favourite films at home.
19. Get a celebration buddy, someone who is specifically there for the reason of sharing celebrations with, and then DM or voice note to share your celebration in real time.
20. Create a celebration wishlist for motivation and then treat yourself to something on it when you next celebrate.

What other ideas can you come up with for everyday celebration as you take action toward your BIG, BOLD, BEAUTIFUL soul goals and reach key stages of your BIG, BOLD, BEAUTIFUL journey? List them out below:

....

....

....

ACTIVATING YOUR DISCO BALL HEART THROUGH GRATITUDE –
THE ULTIMATE ACT OF LOVE FOR YOUR BIG, BOLD, BEAUTIFUL LIFE

Great! So you've explored the power of celebration, and even how you are going to bring celebration into your BIG, BOLD, BEAUTIFUL journey; now let's go a little deeper.

When you strip everything back, your BIG, BOLD, BEAUTIFUL life is one lived in love. Being so fully and completely in love with a BIG, BOLD, BEAUTIFUL life that is true to you. People who have gone through near death experiences, or have shared about life lessons from their death beds, talk about the power of unconditional love in a life well-lived.

Being in love with your BIG, BOLD, BEAUTIFUL life means bringing in the power of gratitude for everything you already have, everything you are creating – to *you* and what you came here to do. Why? Because all of that love and gratitude is emotion, and emotion is energy in motion. This energy in motion operates at a vibrational frequency, which you get to be an energetic match for as you create and live your BIG, BOLD, BEAUTIFUL life.

And the frequency of gratitude and celebration? 540MHz, one of the highest vibrations you can be in resonance with, which also happens to be the frequency of love.

By making time for gratitude and celebration you increase the energetic frequency for your BIG, BOLD, BEAUTIFUL life from a foundational place of love. Gratitude is the energy of love that gives that empowered plan and vision the perfect conditions in which to grow and thrive.

In the final exercise of the final step of our BIG, BOLD, BEAUTIFUL adventure through the pages of this book, you will find a wonderful gratitude practice that will increase the energetic vibration on this incredible journey of love.

EXERCISE

BIG, BOLD, BEAUTIFUL GRATITUDE PRACTICE

I've got my friend, and brave business coach, Caroline Thompson to thank for sharing this simple and powerful gratitude practice with me, created by lifestyle coach Bekie Eakins. Caroline and I share this daily practice of simple gratitude with each other. It's a beautiful way to raise the energy of celebration in every day, to hear the magic of what we are bringing into BIG, BOLD, BEAUTIFUL existence, and be present to all the BIG, BOLD, BEAUTIFUL things we already have.

You can do this on your own as a daily practice, but to take it to the next level you can do it with another person or a small group of trusted friends, who will be open to receiving the gifts of this simple and significant process. Sharing your voice and receiving the energy of gratitude makes it even more powerful; what we say, we create. Harnessing the energy of gratitude for your BIG, BOLD, BEAUTIFUL vision puts it into turbo charge!

THE SET-UP

Gather your soul crew. This should be a group of between 2 and 4 people who are willing to commit 5–10 minutes of each day to the gratitude practice.

Set up a messaging group, where you can share voice notes with each other.

THE PROCESS

1. Share two minutes of gratitude.

In a voice note share two minutes of as many things that you can find to be grateful for right now.

The reason that you need to share two minutes or more of gratitude is that you get to look beyond the obvious for what you're grateful for. It helps you to see the true BIG, BOLD, BEAUTIFUL magic that already exists in your life.

2. Spend one minute talking about your day ahead.

Share this minute talking about your day as if it has already happened and you are grateful for all the amazing things that have happened within it.

This creates the pathways for activating your BIG, BOLD, BEAUTIFUL vision and soul goals. Sharing gratitude from a place of intention brings it into the present moment as if it's already in existence. This is also a great opportunity to set the energetic tone for your day ahead.

Example: "I am grateful for a day which was full of calm and ease, yet brimming with fun and connection."

3. Spend one minute talking about your future.

Spend a minute sharing gratitudes you have for your future, again as if they have already happened, and feel the power of how you feel in your body and what your energy feels like when the things you are creating for your BIG, BOLD, BEAUTIFUL life have been birthed.

This is a gorgeous way to create the energetic and embodied anchor points for the things you are bringing into existence. Try to make this as much of a sensory experience as you can so that your mind and body bring everything into aligned action to make them happen.

Example: "I am sitting in a peaceful room in my beautiful new home surrounded by pictures and objects that make me feel happy. I have my favourite incense burning and filling the room with its delicious scent as I look out over our garden. The sun is shining and I can hear the birds singing away. I am grateful for the time I have as I drink tea out of my favourite mug. I can feel the smooth surface of the mug as it keeps my hands warm. I love that I get to take this precious time each day to think about what I am creating and working on this week. I am so grateful that I created a work pattern based around my own energy and needs."

4. Listen to your soul crew's gratitudes.

Listening to your soul crew's gratitudes will help boost that flow of positive celebratory energy for you. It gets multiplied within the group, and will serve as inspiration for your gratitude practice, each and every day.

You will find that as you share and witness gratitudes on a daily basis, the more you find to be grateful for in your BIG, BOLD, BEAUTIFUL life, and you have your own, and your soul crew's dreams and visions witnessed and shared.

STEP SEVEN REVIEW TIME

I hope you have loved this step in our BIG, BOLD, BEAUTIFUL adventure together as much as I have. It's been an energetic high five to everything that's in play now for your BIG, BOLD, BEAUTIFUL life. It puts the BIG, the BOLD and the BEAUTIFUL into every aspect of this journey – the creation of your BIG, BOLD BEAUTIFUL vision, the action toward your soul goals, and the rewriting and reprogramming of brain, body, behaviours and narratives to be in energetic alignment to support you on your journey … all of it!

Exploring celebration is exploring a life-enhancing commitment to everything that is BIG, BOLD and BEAUTIFUL. Actioning that celebration is fundamental to your ongoing and sustainable success.

Before you turn these final few pages, let's recap on STEP SEVEN and the POWER OF SELF-CELEBRATION. Here's a review of what you've explored, and what you can come back to time and time again.

Here's how to harness the power of celebration:

✓ Create your *loving self-acceptance celebration practice* by celebrating and powering up your strengths and observing your "weaknesses" in relation to your soul goals to learn and take empowered action as you move forward.

✓ Power up your everyday with *self-celebration* so you can become your own cheerleader and create a vibrational shift that's in alignment with your BIG, BOLD, BEAUTIFUL goals and vision.

✓ Explore *20 ideas for everyday celebration* to put power to the small wins that will give your brain and body the tools to increase your capacity for receiving more BIG, BOLD, BEAUTIFUL good stuff.

✓ Light up your disco ball heart, with the powerful *daily gratitude practice*. It's the ultimate act of love and manifestation to bring your BIG, BOLD, BEAUTIFUL vision into embodied being.

Here we are, at the finish line and on the final step of kickstarting your BIG, BOLD, BEAUTIFUL life.

What a ride this has been, learning how to ignite the energetic confetti cannons and pop the champagne corks, as you take steps and actions on this BIG, BOLD, BEAUTIFUL journey.

As we draw a glorious, BIG, BOLD, BEAUTIFUL close to this step, I am celebrating you.

Here's to your BIG, BOLD, BEAUTIFUL life.
Here's to your disco ball heart, shining wildly and brightly.
Here's to you.

Before you close these pages, and get going with everything you've been practising putting into play, head over for one last BIG, BOLD, BEAUTIFUL breakout ritual. This time, you are going to discover a wonderful practice of creating a gratitude ceremony, to honour everything you are creating with a heart full of thanks and love.

BREAKOUT RITUAL
NATURE GRATITUDE CEREMONY
(DESPACHO)

In this final BIG, BOLD, BEAUTIFUL breakout ritual I'm sharing one of my absolute favourites; a gratitude ceremony. I bring this practice in some form or another to every workshop, retreat and programme I host. There's something so special about sharing your appreciation for everything you have in your life with others. Having a space for gratitude and mutual celebration of all things BIG, BOLD and BEAUTIFUL, is like having all the mirrors on our collective disco ball hearts lighting up and shining off of one another. True energetic vibration in action.

There are endless ways you can practise gratitude and create ritual around it. This one, the Despacho ceremony, was shared with me as part of my Qoya training with Rochelle Schieck in the jungles of Costa Rica. I was grateful for every moment of that experience, I can tell you. Rochelle learned this practice from the Q'ero, an ancient shamanic community in Peru. It was here that she learned and participated in daily ceremonies where the Q'ero show their reverence and thanks for *Pachamama* (Mother Earth). The Quechan word for this ceremony is "Hariweequi", which means to "offer with one's own hand". The more commonly used name is "despacho", which is Spanish for "to send". The despacho is a powerful way to "dispatch" your gratitude and celebrations for each step of your BIG, BOLD, BEAUTIFUL journey by connecting to nature.

Despachos can be created anytime and anywhere. They work well in a group and can be practised solo too. The idea is to create an offering of thanks, which you gift back to Mother Earth to be in "Ayni" – the right relationship – between nature with you and around you.

This is a simplified version of how to conduct a despacho. Should you wish to delve deeper into the indigenous ritual, as taught by the Q'ero, I highly recommend it.

What you will need for your despacho (gratitude ceremony):

- A large piece of paper that will form the base of your gratitude parcel / bundle.
- Some string to tie your bundle together once completed.
- Earth offerings to add to the despacho ...
  - Three leaves to make a *Qintu*, which forms your intention prayers.
  - Anything biodegradable that you would like to add to your gratitude bundle ...
    - Flowers/leaves/pinecones
    - Nuts/seeds/beans/pulses/rice/grains
    - Cacao/chocolate

- o Herbs/spices
- o Incense

As this is a gratitude offering for Mother Earth it's always good to find earth offerings that come from the land that you are on. Your despacho bundle is gifted back to the Earth, once you've shared your gratitude, so it's important that everything you use is biodegradable.

1. *Prepare your despacho.*

Place the paper flattened out in front of you, or in the centre if you're in a group.

2. *Gather your earth offerings.*

Place the offerings in bowls, around the outside of what is to become your despacho.

3. *Create sacred space.*

This is a moment of contemplation to bring reverence to the ceremony. You may want to light a candle, burn a smudge stick or incense, say a prayer, sing, chant or meditate.

4. *Create intention with your Qintu.*

Gather the three leaves you have collected for your Qintu into a fan shape in your hand. Set your intention for the despacho by blowing in your gratitude and blessings for Mother Nature and the Earth into the leaves. Do this three times. Make sure everyone around the despacho has blown their intentions into the leaves.

5. *Place the leaves of the Qintu in a circle into the despacho.*

This will form the base on which you will place your earth offerings.

6. *Start to add the gifts of your gratitude to the despacho.*

Each person takes a turn to take some of the earth offerings from the bowls around the despacho. Take some of the offerings from the bowls into the palm of your hand, bring them to your heart, share what you are grateful for and giving thanks for. Blow your thanks into the offerings in your hands and then add to the centre of the bundle. Then, the next person takes the offering into their hands, gives thanks and blows into the offering before offering to the bundle. Continue so that everyone has a chance to share. This doesn't have to go in order. The idea is that, as gratitude comes into each person's heart, they share from that place.

Take your time. The Q'ero can take up to two hours to complete their gratitude. The idea is that you can carry on saying "thank you" until you could go on saying it for ever.

7. *Once complete, invite everyone to close their eyes.*

Listen in to receive any messages that come from this beautiful practice. Stay open and curious. If you would like to say one last "thank you" to Pachamama and the Earth, now is the time.

8. *Wrap your despacho bundle.*

Take your string and wrap your earth offering into a parcel or bundle.

9. *Release the despacho back to spirit.*

There are three ways to transform the energy of the despacho bundle and give it back to Mother Earth. Similar to the elements release rituals you learned about in the breakout ritual at the end of STEP THREE, you can burn your gratitude bundle for rapid transformation, or you can bury it for slow release, or release it into water for purification.

This brings your gratitude ceremony to a close. It's a beautiful ritual to really help you take your time to anchor your gratitude for, and at, each step of your BIG, BOLD, BEAUTIFUL journey.

CONCLUSION

Here we are, you brave and bold soul seeker. While we may be at the end of this exploration together, this is never really the end … simply another beginning.

You see, every time you step onto the curiosity quest for living a BIG, BOLD, BEAUTIFUL life, you are learning and growing, which always brings with it new beginnings … new explorations … new experiences in life, love and everything in between …

And the truth of it all is, that your BIG, BOLD, BEAUTIFUL journey is for life, not just in the pages of this seven-step guide. What you have uncovered about your life and yourself throughout this book is just the tip of the iceberg.

My hope is that what you've begun to reveal for yourself throughout the seven steps opens you up to a whole voyage of discovery, taking you on epic quests throughout your BIG, BOLD, BEAUTIFUL life. Quests that take you into unexplored territories and open up treasure chests of wisdom for you and your BIG, BOLD, BEAUTIFUL vision. Ones that activate passion and purpose within everything you do, and get that disco ball heart of yours shining brightly with everything that you are here to be.

This does come with fair warning: once you open up that cupboard of curiosities and step on through, you will never turn back. I know from my own personal experience that it's something that is never complete. There is always more to learn and more to discover, but that's the glorious part of the BIG, BOLD, BEAUTIFUL adventure.

That's why there's always more to delve into within the seven steps. This book was never designed to be read once and left sitting on a shelf. It's here as an active tour guide every time you set off on an expedition into the wild unknown of your BIG, BOLD, BEAUTIFUL life.

Every time a purpose-fuelled idea is sparked … head to STEPS ONE and TWO to Create the Vision and get a plan of action in place, so you can Find Your Focus.

Every time you find yourself in that sticky place of doubt and overwhelm, head to STEP THREE and bring out the BIG, BOLD, BEAUTIFUL exercises and guidance to Bust Beyond Resistance.

Come back to STEP FOUR to Dial Up Your Energy to get in alignment and connected to all that incredible wisdom you have within you to create the juice for the journey.

Activate all your good stuff by delving into STEPS FIVE and SIX for all the Self-Empowerment and Self-Care mastery that will help you feel invigorated as you take flight on your BIG, BOLD, BEAUTIFUL vision quest.

And then celebrate it all in STEP SEVEN as I am celebrating all that you are, and all you are here to be.

What a freaking gift it all is.

What a freaking gift you are.

I'm excited for you.

What a BIG, BOLD, BEAUTIFUL ride this has been. And it's only just begun.

Whatever you do, and wherever you go from this point forward, I'm here for the ride! Do come and share the magical adventures of your BIG, BOLD, BEAUTIFUL life with me. I'll be ready with the disco balls and pom poms as you do.

Instagram: katetaylorcreativeliving

Facebook: katetaylorcreativeliving

CONCLUSION

If you would like to take everything you've experienced within this book, and experience it with me, and a soul crew of people who will become friends for life, you can find out more about the Kickstart Your BIG, BOLD, BEAUTIFUL Life programme, at www.katetaylor.co.

BIG, BOLD, BEAUTIFUL REFERENCES

STEP TWO: FIND YOUR FOCUS

National Institute of General Medical Sciences, Circadian Rhythms: https://nigms.nih.gov/education/fact-sheets/Pages/circadian-rhythms.aspx.

Individual Variation and the Genetics of Sleep, Harvard Medical School: http://healthysleep.med.harvard.edu/healthy/science/variations/individual-variation-genetics#:~:text=The%20circadian%20rhythms%20generated%20by, determined%E2%80%94at%20least%20in%20part.

Lunsford-Avery, J. R. and Kollins, S. H. Editorial Perspective: Delayed circadian rhythm phase: a cause of late-onset attention-deficit/hyperactivity disorder among adolescents? J Child Psychol Psychiatry. 2018 Dec;59(12):1248-1251. doi: 10.1111/jcpp.12956. Epub 2018 Sep 3. PMID: 30176050; PMCID: PMC6487490.

Kleitman N. Basic rest-activity cycle–22 years later. Sleep. 1982;5(4):311–7. doi: 10.1093/sleep/5.4.311. PMID: 6819628.

STEP THREE: BUST BEYOND RESISTANCE

Pelletier, K. R. Mind-body health: research, clinical, and policy applications. Am J Health Promot. 1992 May-Jun;6(5):345-58. doi: 10.4278/0890-1171-6.5.345. PMID: 10148755.

Hernandez, R., Bassett, S. M., Boughton, S. W., Schuette, SA., Shiu, E. W., & Moskowitz, J. T. (2018). Psychological Well-Being and Physical Health: Associations, Mechanisms, and Future Directions. Emotion Review, 10(1), 18–29: https://doi.org/10.1177/1754073917697824.

Nummenmaa, L., Glerean, E., Hari, R. and Hietanen, J. K. (2013). Bodily maps of emotions. 111 (2) 646-651: https://doi.org/10.1073/pnas.1321664111.

Shaffer, J. Neuroplasticity and Clinical Practice: Building Brain Power for Health, (2016). doi:10.3389/fpsyg.2016.01118 Retrieved from https://www.frontiersin.org/articles/10.3389/fpsyg.2016.01118.

STEP FOUR: DIAL UP YOUR BIG, BOLD, BEAUTIFUL ENERGY

Soosalu, G., Henwood, S. and Deo, A. Head, heart, and gut in decision making: development of a multiple brain Preference Questionnaire: https://journals.sagepub.com/doi/10.1177/2158244019837439.

Soosalu, G. and Henwood, S. The Three Brains of Leadership: Harnasing the Wisdom Within: https://www.researchgate.net/publication/274699861_The_three_brains_of_Leadership_Harnasing_the_Wisdom_within.

Sonnenburg, J. and Sonnenburg, E. (2015, May 1). Gut Feelings – the "Second Brain" in Our Gastrointestinal Systems (Excerpt). Retrieved from: https://www.scientificamerican.com/article/gut-feelings-the-second-brain-in-our-gastrointestinal-systems-excerpt/.

Howland, R. Vagus Nerve Stimulation: https://www.ncbi.nlm.nih.gov/pmc/articles/PMC4017164/.

Brown, S. J. What the vagus nerve is and how to stimulate it for better mental health: https://www.forbes.com/sites/womensmedia/2021/04/15/what-the-vagus-nerve-is-and-how-to-stimulate-it-for-better-mental-health/?sh=10603c0f6250.

Breit, S., Kupferberg, A., Rogler, G and Hasler, G. Vagus Nerve as Modulator of the Brain – Gut Axis in Psychiatric and Inflammatory Disorders. Retrieved from: https://www.frontiersin.org/articles/10.3389/fpsyt.2018.00044/full.

Rozanski, A., Bavishi, C., Kubzansky, L. D., Cohen, R. Association of Optimism With Cardiovascular Events and All-Cause

Mortality: A Systematic Review and Meta-analysis. Retrieved from: https://jamanetwork.com/journals/jamanetworkopen/fullarticle/2752100.

STEP FIVE: CREATE A SELF-EMPOWERMENT TOOLKIT

Sathyanarayana Rao, T. S., Asha, M. R., Jagannatha Rao, K. S. and Vasudevaraju, P. The biochemistry of belief. Retrieved from the National Library of Medicine: https://www.ncbi.nlm.nih.gov/pmc/articles/PMC2802367/.

Okimoto, T. G., Wenzel, M. and Hedrick, K. Refusing to apologize can have psychological benefits. The European Journal of Social Psychology. Retrieved from: https://www.researchgate.net/publication/264695556_Refusing_to_apologize_can_have_psychological_benefits_and_we_issue_no_mea_culpa_for_this_research_finding.

Glazier, B. L., & Alden, L. E. (2019). Social anxiety disorder and memory for positive feedback. Journal of Abnormal Psychology, 128(3), 228–233. https://doi.org/10.1037/abn0000407.

Warren, R., Smeets, E. And Neff K. Self-criticism and self-compassion: risk and resilience: being compassionate to oneself is associated with emotional resilience and psychological well-being. Retrieved from: https://self-compassion.org/wp-content/uploads/2016/12/Self-Criticism.pdf.

Sugawara, S. K., Tanaka, S. Okazaki, S., Watanabe, K. and Sadato, N. Social Rewards Enhance Offline Improvements in Motor Skill. Retrieved from: https://doi.org/10.1371/journal.pone.0048174.

Pluut, H., and Wonders, J. (2020). Not able to lead a healthy life when you need it the most: Dual role of lifestyle behaviors in the association of blurred work-life boundaries with well-being. Retrieved from: https://doi.org/10.3389/fpsyg.2020.607294.

STEP SIX: HONOUR YOUR SELF-CARE

Mansfield, L., Daykin. N., and Kay. T. Leisure and wellbeing, Leisure Studies (2020), Retrieved from: https://doi.org/10.10 80/02614367.2020.1713195.

Oberste M, de Waal P, Joisten N, Walzik D, Egbringhoff M, Javelle F, Bloch W, Zimmer P. Acute aerobic exercise to recover from mental exhaustion - a randomized controlled trial. Physiol Behav. 2021 Nov 1;241:113588. doi: 10.1016/j. physbeh.2021.113588. Epub 2021 Sep 11. PMID: 34516957.

World Health Organization (WHO) International Classification of Diseases 11th Revision https://icd.who.int/en/.

Barker, S. Burnt Out: The exhausted person's six-step guide to thriving in a fast-paced world, Aster, 2021.

Bönstrup, M et al. A Rapid Form of Offline Consolidation in Skill Learning. Current Biology, Volume 29, Issue 8, 1346 - 1351.e4.

Asp M. Rest: A Health-Related Phenomenon and Concept in Caring Science. Glob Qual Nurs Res. 2015 Retrieved from: https://www.ncbi.nlm.nih.gov/pmc/articles/PMC5342845/.

Lamp, A., Cook, M. Soriano Smith, R. N., Belenky, B. Exercise, nutrition, sleep, and waking rest? Sleep, Volume 42, Issue 10, October 2019, zsz138, Retreived from: https://doi. org/10.1093/sleep/zsz138.

Marshall-Pescini, S., Schaebs, F. S., Gaugg, A., Meinert, A., Deschner, T., Range, F. The Role of Oxytocin in the Dog – Owner Relationship. Animals 2019, 9(10), 792. https://doi. org/10.3390/ani9100792.

Schmuck D. Does Digital Detox Work? Exploring the Role of Digital Detox Applications for Problematic Smartphone Use and Well-Being of Young Adults Using Multigroup Analysis. Cyberpsychol Behav Soc Netw. 2020 Aug;23(8):526-532. doi: 10.1089/cyber.2019.0578. Epub 2020 Apr 30. PMID: 32354288.

El-Khoury J, Haidar R, Kanj RR, Bou Ali L, Majari G. Characteristics of social media 'detoxification' in university students. Libyan J Med. 2021 Dec;16(1):1846861. doi: 10.1080/19932820.2020.1846861. PMID: 33250011; PMCID: PMC7717533.

STEP SEVEN: HARNESS THE POWER OF SELF-CELEBRATION

Wood, A. M., Maltby, J., Gillett, R., Linley, P. A. and Joseph, S. (2008) The role of gratitude in the development of social support, stress, and depression: two longitudinal studies. Journal of Research in Personality, Volume 42 (4). pp. 854-871. doi:10.1016/j.jrp.2007.11.003.

Bono, G., Emmons, R and Mccullough, M. (2012). Gratitude in Practice and the Practice of Gratitude. 10.1002/9780470939338. ch29. Retrieved from: https://www.researchgate.net/publication/279403394_Gratitude_in_Practice_and_the_Practice_of_Gratitude.

Glaser, J. E. (2015, December). Celebration time. Psychology Today. Retrieved from https://www.psychologytoday.com/us/blog/conversational-intelligence/201512/celebration-time.

Emmons, R. Thanks!: How Practicing Gratitude Can Make You Happier, 2008, HarperOne.

Amabile, T. M. and Kramer, S. J., 2011. The power of small wins. Harvard Business Review, 89(5), pp.70-80.

Gable, S. and Haidt, J. (2005). What (and Why) Is Positive Psychology?. Review of General Psychology. 9. 10.1037/1089-2680.9.2.103.

Ellis, R.D. and Newton, N.: Consciousness & Emotion: Agency, conscious choice, and selective perception, 2005, John Benjamin Publishing Company.

Hill, P. L., Allemand, M., Roberts, B. W. Examining the Pathways between Gratitude and Self-Rated Physical Health across Adulthood. Pers Individ Dif. 2013 Jan;54(1):92-96. doi: 10.1016/j.paid.2012.08.011. PMID: 23139438; PMCID: PMC3489271.

Muehsam D and Ventura C. Life rhythm as a symphony of oscillatory patterns: electromagnetic energy and sound vibration modulates gene expression for biological signaling and healing. Glob Adv Health Med. 2014 Mar;3(2):40-55. doi: 10.7453/gahmj.2014.008. PMID: 24808981; PMCID: PMC4010966.

ACKNOWLEDGEMENTS

Thank you to all my friends and family who've been there for me all the way through the process of bringing these words to life. Your belief and encouragement means everything. The biggest of thanks is to you Si, for your love and steadfast support, which may not seem much to you, but it means the absolute world to me.

To Matt Taylor – my brother from another mother – for being the conduit of so much on this journey of personal and spiritual development, and whizzing me around Barcelona on the back of a scooter for my first book writing in the BIG, BOLD, BEAUTIFUL city of Barcelona! It had to start somewhere, and I can't think of a better person, or place, to do that with.

To Beth Bishop, Rachel Gregory, and all the team at Welbeck. Beth, thank you for taking a chance and seeing that "something more" in me and my work. I've learned so much about connecting deeper to my work through your guidance. And to Rachel for taking my words – and often long-winded, "jazz hands" sentences – and making it all flow and make sense! This book is so much better for both of your guiding hands.

To all of my teachers along the path who've held space and showed me what's possible when you open the door of curiosity to delve deeper into this thing called life. In particular, Rochelle Schieck for the offering of Qoya inspired movement, as the conduit to so much of what has brought the words and learnings in this book and inside of me out and into BIG, BOLD, BEAUTIFUL being.

The Q'ero people for their teachings and the blessing for the despacho ceremony to be shared. And to all indigenous people and teachers for your cultures and traditions that have been such a beautiful gift to this book and to our learnings. I thank you for your generosity of heart and spirit.

To all my clients who've inspired every word in this book. I write this book with the wisdom of each and everyone woven into each line.

And the biggest of all glitter cannons has to go to all the disco ball soul crew who've braved the adventure in the Kickstart Your BIG, BOLD, BEAUTIFUL Life Programme. Thank you for allowing me to be the custodian and dreamcatcher for your BIG, BOLD, BEAUTIFUL visions. Every unfurling, every step, every brave move, every share, every tear, every belly laugh has lit up this disco ball heart of mine. Here's to all the friendships forged, and adventures explored.

Here's to many more.